The Commodity of Care
Home Care Reform in Ontario

Edited by Paul Leduc Browne

Canadian Centre for Policy Alternatives

Copyright © 2003

All rights reserved. No part of this book may be reproduced or transmitted in any form or by any means, electronic or mechanical, including photocopying, or by any information storage or retrieval system, without permission in writing from the publishers or the author.

The contents of this book are the opinions of its authors and do not necessarily reflect the views of the Board of Directors or members of the Canadian Centre for Policy Alternatives.

National Library of Canada Cataloguing in Publication

The commodity of care : home care reform in Ontario / edited by Paul Leduc Browne.

Includes bibliographical references.
ISBN 0-88627-271-8

1. Home care services—Ontario. I. Browne, Paul Leduc II. Canadian Centre for Policy Alternatives. III. Title.

RA645.37.C3C65 2003   362.1'4'09713   C2003-906309-7

Printed and bound in Canada

Published by

Canadian Centre for Policy Alternatives
Suite 410, 75 Albert Street
Ottawa, ON K1P 5E7
Tel 613-563-1341   Fax 613-233-1458
http://www.policyalternatives.ca
ccpa@policyalternatives.ca

Contents

Acknowledgements i

Introduction
The Social Division of Care in a World of Commodities
Paul Leduc Browne 1

Chapter 1
Caregiving in Historical Perspective
Pat Armstrong and Olga Kits 23

Chapter 2
Responding to State Retrenchment: An Historical Perspective on Non-Profit Home Health and Social Care in Ontario
Tamara J. Daly 65

Chapter 3
The Welfare State in Retreat: The Impact of Home-Care Restructuring on Women's Labour
Allison Williams 121

Chapter 4
Offloading the Cost of Home Care: The Impact on Front-Line Workers and Agencies
Denise O'Connor 147

Chapter 5
Care, Power, and Commodification
Paul Leduc Browne 171

Contributors 213

Acknowledgements

I would like to thank the Social Sciences and Humanities Research Council of Canada for a strategic research grant which made possible the editing and publication of this book. My own chapters in the book stem from projects generously supported by the Social Sciences and Humanities Research Council and Human Resources Development Canada. The book was a long time in production and I would like to thank its authors not only for their excellent contributions, but also for their patience and forbearance. I would like to thank Pascale Houle, Nadia Lauzon, Marie-Ève Lavoie, Gabriela Lopez, Abdollah Payrow Shabani, and David Welch for their invaluable assistance with various aspects of the research and production of the book. Kerri-Anne Finn (as always) did a fine job laying out the text and was such a pleasure to work with. Thanks to Studio 2 for the great cover. I am very grateful to Melanie Allison, Ansky Espinosa, Bruce Campbell, Ed Finn, Erika Shaker, and Diane Touchette for all of their support. Many thanks to the reviewers who read the manuscripts of the chapters, and provided constructive criticism and sound advice.

Paul Leduc Browne

Introduction
The Social Division of Care in a World of Commodities
Paul Leduc Browne

> **Commodity** n. L/ME. [(O)Fr. *commodité* or L. *commoditas*,
> f. *commodus*: see prec., -ITY.]
> I 1 Suitability; fitting utility; convenience, as a property of some-
> thing. 2a A person's convenience. b (An) advantage, (a) benefit; (self-
> ish) interest. c Expediency. d Profit, gain. 3 Opportunity, occasion.
> II 4 A thing of use or value; spec. a thing that is an object of trade,
> esp. a raw material or an agricultural crop. b A thing one deals in or
> makes use of. 5 A quantity of wares; spec. one lent on credit by a
> usurer for resale, usu. to the usurer himself. (Brown, 452)
> Related term: the commode.

The Social Division of Care

If the study of tools can reconstruct a lost culture, a future archaeol-
ogy of home care might well centre on the commode. A simple bench
opening over an attached bucket, the commode is a mobile toilet.
Thanks to the commode, the toilet can be brought to us when we
have lost the power to walk to it. Its name derives from its very commodity, its "fitting utility" and "convenience."

The French monarch Louis XIV famously used such a device, a
chaise percée. In the pageantry built around the Sun King's person,
attendance on each of his bodily functions had become a high honour
surrounded by elaborate ceremony. His excretions were a moment of
public solemnity. Not only could Louis XIV command the caring
attention of his subjects; proximity to his very excrement had become
a high honour.

Today, our basic bodily functions, though a matter of elementary
need, are nonetheless very private, indeed surrounded by shame, eu-

phemism, and silence—and much the same can be said for the activity that surrounds them: carework. This type of work is complex and multifaceted, but it is first and foremost bodywork. (Twigg, 2000a) For example, in home care, workers confront the body's materiality in its immediacy, in the form of bodily wastes and fluids. These aspects tend to be eclipsed by the bland euphemisms to which we all resort when discussing these matters. As Julia Twigg puts it, bodywork, the labour of tending to another's body, "verges on areas of taboo in connection with sexuality and human waste."

In his satirical poem, "L'éclipse," Jacques Prévert writes that the Sun King one night sat on his *chaise percée*—and disappeared! Indeed, gone today is the aura that made the monarch's very excretions an object of reverence. Gone, too, is the courtly honour that surrounded the care provided him. Carework today is either concealed in the privacy of the home or of an institution, or, if public, clothed in rituals and other trappings that enable those who perform it to distance themselves from it: "[It] is potentially demeaning work, and when undertaken by high-status individuals it is typically accompanied by distancing techniques." (Twigg, 2000b, 391)

To be sure, the pageantry surrounding Louis XIV's person constituted precisely such distancing techniques; at the same time, by involving members of the nobility in tending to his most basic bodily needs, the Sun King also cemented their subordination to his person. However, where the monarch made his most powerful subjects tend to his personal needs, relations between today's caregivers and care recipients are far more variable. Much bodywork is now performed within specialized institutions (e.g., hospitals or diagnostic clinics), where a range of technical procedures may be carried out on individuals, in a more or less impersonal way, by orders of men and women wielding esoteric knowledge like a modern priesthood. Such events display all of the elements of ritual: technicians dressed in masks and uniforms (lab coats, scrubs), rooms designed and furnished in extraordinary fashion (e.g., x-ray labs or operating rooms—which are even referred to in the U.K. as "operating theatres"). Even those who must deal with bodily fluids and wastes wear latex gloves as a distancing medium. In such institutions, the care recipient tends to be a *patient*—etymologically, one who suffers, to whom things are done.

The distancing techniques, media and rituals are also a way of representing and displaying authority: that of the seventeenth-century state embodied in the absolute monarch—and that of the hospital, no longer embodied in this or that individual, but in the very institution as a place of Knowledge. The Sun King's very person embodied visible, overwhelming power, justified through the invocation of his divine right to wield it. The medical institution's power, however, draws its legitimacy from its scientific neutrality and objectivity, from its appearance of transcending the political, of hardly constituting *power* as such. Like Louis XIV in Prévert's poem, the political dimension of the labour of care has been eclipsed by social taboos and the ideology of scientific authority.

When care is provided in non-institutional settings, for example in the home, the power dynamics can be quite different. Thus, it is not enough to contemplate the tool on its own. The commode is brought to us, or we to it. It is used with the help of another. *The key question, then, is what social relationship binds the commode's user to that helper.* It is a relationship centered on labour, a relation of production.

If home care is a form of labour, it is purposive activity (Lukács, 1980, 3). Each and every labour process is initiated by the setting of some purpose to be achieved, some goal to be attained. It requires effecting some transformation of the material—both physical and social—world, in order to bring some new reality into being. And it results in the production or reproduction of new or existing physical and social conditions (instruments, physical states—e.g., health, cleanliness—, social relationships). All work is also social in nature. In analyzing it, we must therefore explore the social relationships that arise within and as a result of it. The answers to three questions determine the nature of these relations of production: Who defines the goal(s)? Who performs the work? Who appropriates the product(s)? Who suffers? Who benefits?

In home care, care recipients, family or other informal caregivers, non-profit organizations, private for-profit businesses, and the state all have a say—but an unequal one—in defining the goals to be achieved and the means to be employed in doing so. The Commission on the Future of Health Care in Canada has defined public health care as a *moral* economy, an economy based on need and solidarity, rather than profit and competition; but, as the Commission also points out, health care is a *mixed* economy. (Romanow, 2002) In today's Ontario, the social division of labour in *home care*—what I call the *social division of care*—is a hybrid of three fundamental economic logics: reciprocity, state redistribution, and profit accumulation. (Laville, 2001, 1994, 1993; Laville & Eme, 1999) We can further observe a division between formal and informal, waged and unwaged, professional and unprofessional labour, as well as between the production of standardizable and relational "services." (Laville & Nyssens, 2001; Leys, 2001) The appropriate form of these divisions of care is at the heart of this book.

These questions have been forced on to the political and research agenda by the substantial public policy changes that have occurred since 1996, when Ontario's Conservative government introduced a form of *managed competition* to home care, an experiment without precedent in Canadian health care. Under managed competition:

- the provincial government set home care policy and overall budget envelopes;
- the power of allocating public monies and selecting provider agencies was vested in forty-three territorially based, formally autonomous corporations[1], the Community Care Access Centres (CCACs);
- the CCACs were responsible for co-ordination, assessment and case management;
- they were obliged to contract with outside agencies for service provision (shift nursing, home support, occupational therapy, etc.);
- they followed a formal procedure for tendering services, receiving and sorting bids, and selecting winners;
- competition was open to both non-profit and for-profit agencies.

Managed competition encompassed areas of production already staffed by waged workers, such as nursing, personal support, physiotherapy, and so on. Forms of care essentially provided by volunteers (e.g., friendly visiting, meals on wheels, congregate dining) continued to be financed directly by the Ministry of Health and Long-Term Care on a fee-for-service basis.

These reforms have changed the face of home care. Many of the agencies and workers that once worked in the sector have left or been forced out, while others have moved in, or come from the margins to capture a large share of the new market. This process has not been smooth; the home-care labour market has seen considerable disruption in several parts of the province. Managed competition has also coincided with the massive shift of patients from hospitals to the home and the significant medicalization of home care. These processes have transformed the division of labour and the way caregiving takes place in the home. Although the contributors to this book do not share a single analysis of home-care reform, they are all critical about the commodification of care implied by managed competition, concluding from their respective studies that it has had and will have a damaging effect on caregivers, care recipients, and the very process of care itself.

There are few comprehensive and accessible studies of recent home-care reform in Ontario, despite its magnitude and impact on the province. This book contributes to filling that gap by situating recent changes in a historical, sociological, and political context. The authors hope that the arguments and insights presented here will be of use to academics, advocates, people working in the field, and users of the home-care system.

Exploring the Social Division of Care: Reciprocity

Although most human beings can care for themselves in some ways, everyone also needs the care of others—and needs others for whom to care. Ideally, care is a relationship arising both out of the need *for* care and the need *to* care, in which, in other words, both the "caregiver" and "care recipient" give and receive something. Although we speak of care*giving*, care *recipients* in most cases participate both in the definition of care goals and the enjoyment of the results. (Laville, 2001;

Twigg, 2000) In an *ideal* situation, labouring together to fulfil specific needs (e.g., assistance with bathing, dressing, eating) generates a logic of *reciprocity*: each action by one is a gift to the other, who feels bound in a positive fashion to return the gift, *to give back²*; each finds enjoyment, even fulfilment, in the relationship. (Gagnon & Saillant, 2000)

Sociologists usefully distinguish *primary* from *secondary sociality*. (Caillé, 2001, 188ff.) The former represents social relationships that are an end in themselves, in which we seek others out for who they are, not because relations with them are the means to some ulterior end. Such relationships are necessarily of a personal nature and are built on a specific history of giving and reciprocity. In secondary sociality, by contrast, our relationships with others flow from their function, rank or status in society and are governed by impersonal rules—law, custom, the rules of the marketplace.

In its essence, the *care* relationship must transcend secondary sociality, enter into the realm of primary sociality, and become an end in itself. In such circumstances, the caregiver will seek out the care recipient for the latter's company and presence, not merely in order to fulfil a mandate or a duty. The care recipient will desire the caregiver's presence for itself, not merely because it is the means of being bathed, dressed, and fed. At its core, it cannot be an impersonal relationship.

Home care bridges the divide between primary and secondary sociality. In home care, a stranger is paid a wage to enter a person's home to care for that person in intimate ways. The ensuing relationship is mandated by an authority (government, employer), yet is unique to those individuals; it is governed by general, codified rules of practice and ethical codes, but is inextricably bound up with a personal relationship of trust and respect between two individuals. It is the means to an end, but can become an end in itself.

Care thus implies a complex set of relationships. This complexity is illustrated by the fact that French and German each require at least three words to capture the subtleties of *care*: *soin, souci, amour* and *Pflege, Sorge, Liebe* respectively—that is, care as tending to, as being concerned for, and as loving. When we speak of *health care* or *home care*, we usually have in mind the first meaning—*tending to, soigner, pflegen*. Yet, it is important to realize two things: first, that we are only able to isolate this sense of care *conceptually*, because the division of labour has done so *socially*; and secondly, that notwithstanding this separation, it is terribly difficult for the worker to divorce care as *tending to* a person's needs from *showing concern* for that person and *giving him or her love*. Care is thus a collective activity of the most immediately *material* kind (looking after the most basic bodily needs) inextricably intermingled with *emotional labour*. Despite the almost universal use of the term "health care delivery," care is not in fact an *object* that could be *delivered*. It *coincides with the relationship in which it occurs*.[3]

This definition of care is what sociologists call an *ideal type*, an abstract model constructed as a way of making sense of the real world, but not intended as a concrete portrait of it. Care is never simply a relationship between two individuals in a vacuum. It always takes place in the context of broader social structures—the family, the state, the market—which have their own power dynamics that limit the blossoming of reciprocity. Eighty-five to ninety percent of care in the home is provided by informal caregivers—parents, children, other relatives, friends, neighbours (see Armstrong and Kits in this volume). Yet, the driving force in the evolution of home care resides in the other 10 to 15 percent of care provided by strangers coming into the home and caring for a living, as a *job*.

State Redistribution and the Home-Care Industry

Publicly mandated home care is an important industry in Ontario today. Provincial government funding of home care has undergone considerable growth over the past twenty years, increasing from $ 46 million, or 1 percent of total provincial health-care spending, in 1980, to $ 1,481 million, or 5 percent, in 2000.[4] (Browne, 2000) About three-quarters of provincial home-care spending is transferred to the forty-three Community Care Access Centres. Acting as brokers on behalf of home-care recipients, the latter purchase nursing, home support, therapies, and medical equipment from private and not-for-profit suppliers. (Browne, 2000) The rest of the provincial home-care budget is spent directly by the Ministry of Health and Long-Term Care in supporting community support services, such as meals on wheels, transportation, friendly visits, or telephone reassurance, provided (mostly on a volunteer basis) by some 350 locally based charitable organizations.

The existence and growth of a large, publicly mandated and funded home-care industry meets at least some of the needs of an ageing population, for whom it is desirable—from the standpoint both of money and of health—that the elderly, chronically ill and disabled be able to stay in their homes where appropriate. But the growth of home care in Ontario also reflects the shift of its role from chronic to post-acute care: in recent years, more and more of the activities once carried out in hospitals, nursing homes, and asylums have come to be performed in the community, indeed in the home. The "hospital within the home" is now a major site of "home health care," as post-acute care occupies an ever-greater place next to social care, such as nutrition (meals on wheels, help with grocery shopping), personal care (bathing, grooming, dressing), housekeeping (help with banking and budgeting, cleaning, maintenance work), and transportation (to medical or social appointments).

The shift of care from institutions to the home has meant a significant *transfer of work* (Glazer 1993, 1988) from a mostly waged, as well as largely professional and regulated, workforce, to a mostly non-waged, non-regulated and non-professional one. The latter also bears most of the cost of caregiving (e.g., lost earnings).[5] Informal caregivers provide eighty-five to ninety percent of home care. Fifty percent take time off from their jobs in order to care for others. Forty percent must cope with additional out-of-pocket expenditures. One quarter of Canadian workers provide care of some kind to an elderly person and a further quarter of them provide personal care (feeding, dressing, bathing). The "sandwich generation" has increased from 9.5 to 15 percent of the workforce. (Armstrong & Kits in this volume; Conference Board, 1999; Church, 1999; Armstrong & Armstrong, 1996) Many of these informal caregivers work beside the thousands of waged workers and volunteers hired or recruited by not-for-profit and for-profit agencies often funded by public home-care programs. This has especially been the case as the home has become a substitute for the hospital as a theatre for post-acute health care.

Among the tasks performed in the home, the most technical remain the domain of professionals, such as registered nurses, physiotherapists, occupational therapists, or social workers. These are the tasks in which the relation with the other's body is mediated by the use of technology (i.e., IVs, catheters, bandages, dialysis machines), by bodies of professional knowledge and by codified procedures. At the other end of the spectrum, activities such as toileting, bathing, grooming, and feeding, in which contact with the body is most immediate, have been assigned to personal support workers, who do not benefit from the same status as members of regulated professions. However, their work too is characterized by the standardization of protocols, processes and methods of evaluation.

The work transfer from the hospital to the home is directly related to the downsizing of the hospital system and can be explained by technological change (the possibility of new, less invasive therapies, and new sites of treatment), changes to the production process, cost-cutting in the name of the federal and provincial imperative of deficit and debt reduction, and the drive to privatize health care spearheaded by powerful corporate interests. (Browne & Welch, 2002; Fuller, 2001; Browne, 2000)

Over the past quarter of a century, the perception spread throughout the most industrialized countries that public expenditures, in particular health and social welfare costs, were spiraling out of control (Light, 2001; Light, 1994, 455; O'Connor, 1973). In Canada, high interest rates and falling government revenues led to the steady rise of federal and provincial government deficits over the 1980s and 1990s. Over the course of the 1990s, those governments introduced a variety of austerity measures designed to restore balanced budgets. In particular, the federal government substantially reduced the amount of money it transferred every year to its provincial counterparts. They, in turn, cut their allocations to municipal governments, school boards, hospital boards, and other local and regional authorities.

In health care, costs were reduced in two ways: by making it cheaper to provide care and by not providing it at all. As wages are the major cost in human services, work was shifted to workers earning lower wages (or no wage at all) in the same institutions (e.g., hospitals), in other parts of the health care system (e.g., home care[6]), or outside of the formal system (e.g., the household). Hospitals received the largest share of provincial health-care dollars. It was logical that major efforts would be made to reduce their number. Over the course of the 1990s, the number of hospitals in Ontario dropped by nearly 25 percent, while the number of hospital beds was cut by 30 percent. Patients were discharged from hospital "quicker and sicker," either into the care of professional home-care services, or into that of their family and neighbours. (Browne, 2000)

The Canada Health Act covers provincial hospital-insurance plans. By virtue of this, hospitals cannot refuse to treat a patient admitted by a physician. On the other hand, home care is defined as an "extended health service" not covered by the Canada Health Act. Consequently, provincial authorities do not have the same obligation to provide care in the home as in the hospital. To be sure, the province covers some costs, but the individual may be charged for nursing, medication, homemaking, or medical equipment or supplies. Provincial regulations cap the number of hours of nursing and homemaking a client may receive, as well as the provision of equipment and supplies (e.g., bathroom commodes, walkers). Practice guidelines not written into the regulations establish orders of priority for access to care (e.g., acuity, availability of informal support). The regulations themselves appear to be mainly a cost-containment measure, as their purpose is to define eligibility and its limits, rather than users' rights. (Browne, 2000) A logic of cost-restraint and rationing is intrinsic to home care reform and restructuring.

The enormous growth of home care in a context of public-expenditure restraint has entailed its transformation. Managing the large volume of "clients" has entailed establishing new management structures and rationalizing the workers' use of time. Doing so in a context of public-sector austerity has meant subjecting carework to new measures of accountability. The impact has been felt by the care recipients, the careworkers, and the provider agencies (see Daly, O'Connor, and Williams in this volume), both with respect to the loss of services, wages, jobs and contracts, and to the changing nature of the labour process. Reciprocity is not absent, to be sure; nor is the co-production of care by the care "giver" and care "recipient." But care cannot be unaffected by a context in which a public authority sends armies of workers into thousands of homes throughout the working day with the mandate of carrying out a specified set of repetitive tasks in short, standardized periods of time.

As in health care and social services more generally, deployment of such social energies and resources to assist people in their homes points to a deep reservoir of solidarity in Canada. The waged workers who labour long hours, often for modest wages, to bring help to fellow citizens who may be in great distress, display great courage, devotion and compassion. But when a public authority or private agency divides carework up into different jobs parcelled out to different workers, and when each of the latter must repeat a same set of tasks many times over a day in short time segments, the holistic process of care becomes a sum of discrete services. Irrespective of the qualities and attitudes of the caregiver, carework is something different than it would be in a situation entirely governed by the logic of reciprocity, rather than a process ruled by the logic of redistribution.

The Commodity of Care

Ontario has long had a mixed economy in health care. The public sector shoulders roughly two-thirds of the costs; individuals and households pay for the rest directly or via their private insurance plans. Health care is provided by a variety of actors: independent professionals (e.g., physicians, physiotherapists), non-profit organizations (e.g., hospitals, home-care agencies, long-term-care facilities), private for-profit corporations (e.g., certain medical clinics, laboratories and diagnostic facilities, home-care agencies, long-term-care facilities), volunteers and informal caregivers.

Collaboration between the public and *not-for-profit* sectors in health and social welfare has deep roots in pre-Confederation Ontario. (Maurutto, 2003) However, the relationship between them has gone through many phases. Whereas in an earlier era, public funding enabled non-profit organizations to participate in the identification of social needs and to develop their own independent social welfare goals in addition, in the most recent period non-profits have figured in government programs essentially as sub-contractors providing specific services on behalf of the state. (Daly in this volume; Scott, 2003; Browne, 1996)

Today, care relationships increasingly unfold in the shadow of the market (Browne & Welch, 2002), of the exchange of *commodities*, i.e. things that are not merely *commodious*, but produced for the purpose of being sold. This is true in general, because capitalism is the overwhelmingly dominant economic system in the world today. Few Canadians can subsist independently of the monetary economy; and on average, they derive roughly four-fifths of their monetary income from market sources (profits, wages, rent, interest) (Browne, 1999).

But it is true in particular as well, because the relationship between market, state and social economy is at the heart of the debate over the future of health and social services throughout the world. Over the past few years, Canada has been deluged with an enormous volume of briefs, speeches and editorials advocating the privatization of health care and social services. But Canada is not the only country where this has been happening. The World Bank, the International Monetary Fund, the Organization for Economic Co-operation and Development, and a number of business-backed think tanks and multinational consulting firms have been spreading the gospel of privatization across the globe. (Serré & Pierru, 2001; Saint-Martin, 2001; Martin, 1993)

The kind of health-care privatization advocated in Canada and elsewhere today is often ambiguous about the distinction between the for-profit and not-for-profit sectors. Essentially, however, it refers to the transfer, in whole or in part, of the costs, administration, or delivery of services from the public to the private, *for-profit* sector, or to the adoption by public enterprises and institutions of administrative structures and practices that mimic those of the private sector.[7] (Browne, 2000; Starr, 1990, 1988) Privatization's proponents regard it as the key to achieving the goals of greater efficiency, lower labour costs, enhanced innovation, and freedom of choice, areas in which they hold markets to be superior to the state enterprise.

The subjection of health care to market competition is not, however, without difficulties. As Light points out: "Clinical medicine is rife with uncertainties and too often contingent on diagnosis and response. Thus 'products' often cannot be defined, and property rights may be unclear. Physicians vary substantially in how they treat the same problem. Good market information is poor and highly asymmetrical. The absence of these requirements for beneficial competition can mean that competition is harmful to patients and society." (Light, 2001) Various models of *managed competition* have been presented as solutions combining the best of both worlds—the cost-control and equity-ensuring function of a single payer capable of protecting the public purse and the invididual "client," and the productivity, efficiency, adaptability, and capacity for innovation of the private sector. (Enthoven, 1993, 1988; Light, 2001, 1995, 1993) As Serré and Pierru note, the neo-liberal discourse of international organizations comprises a diagnosis (public health systems' inefficiency), a slogan (managed competition), and therapies drawn from the new public management.[8] Such themes were at the heart of the Harris government's restructuring of the Ontario public sector in the 1990s, in particular in its strategy to reform home care.

Managed competition has injected a new purpose into home care work: the imperative of accumulating and maximizing profit, or at the very least, for non-profits, of maximizing the sale of caring activities. All providers, whether for-profit or non-profit, must reduce costs and generate increasing sales in order to compete in a tight market. Because CCACs pay provider agencies by the visit, the agencies must maximize the number of nursing and home support visits they make. As a result, nurses' work has been reorganized in some agencies to maximize visits, at the expense of nurses' role in planning their care schedules. Workers in some non-profit agencies have faced deteriorating working conditions, e.g., salary freezes, cuts to their benefits and expenses, and increasing part-time work, as a direct result of financial pressures on their employers brought on by managed competition. Non-profit agencies have also revamped and streamlined their administrative and management systems, in order to save money and be more competitive in a sales-oriented environment.

Managed competition appears to have harmed care networks in two fundamental ways. First, trust is essential to the forging of reciprocity, especially in home care, given its intimate nature. The continuity over time of the relationship between caregiver and care recipient is a basic condition in building and maintaining that trust. However, competitive bidding has regularly broken that continuity, as the workers employed by agencies that have lost contracts have been replaced by the staff of the agencies that have won. Secondly, caring agencies thrive within networks characterized by high-trust relationships, mutual support, common values, and knowledge-sharing, as opposed to markets characterized by low-trust relationships, competition, secrecy, divergent interests, and the primacy of financial accountability and control. (Flynn, Williams & Pickard, 1996) Unfortunately, competition has ended or altered the patterns of co-operation between agencies.

Outline of the Book

This book is divided into five chapters. In Chapter One, Pat Armstrong and Olga Kits provide an overview of caregiving: what it is, who provides it, who receives it, how it has changed and how it has remained the same over the last century. They also propose a set of principles to guide policies affecting care. Much of their discussion focuses on unwaged caregivers and considers the conditions and constraints the latter face in striving to work in relationships of reciprocity in social contexts ruled by the logics of state redistribution and market exchange. They argue that people willingly care for others, indeed that "those who receive care now or in the past themselves provide care, and caregiving is often part of rewarding relationships." At the same time, "the demands on caregivers are expanding enormously with the increasing acuity and disability levels of those receiving informal care." Furthermore, "there are more people needing this complex care at the same time as the welfare state is reducing services provided in the formal system and increasing pressures on families in general and women in particular to fill the gaps." This comes at a time when "more and more women have little choice but to work in the labour force, few of their labour force jobs allow them to provide care and, if they do give up full-time paid work in order to care, they are jeopardizing not only their future employment but also their money for old age as well." The consequence is that "this caregiving is often a burden under current conditions, placing strains not only on the health of the providers and recipients but also on their relationships and on both their current and future finances." The authors conclude their chapter with a ten-point framework for assessing legislation, regulations and policies pertaining to care.

Voluntary non-profit organizations could be thought of as the institutional epitome of the logic of reciprocity. But like informal caregivers, they too have always had to operate in a broader society ruled by the market and the state. In Chapter Two, Tamara Daly provides a detailed history of the evolution of the voluntary sector in Ontario's changing home-care-policy environment. She sees four main periods: before 1945, voluntary organizations supported financially by government acted as providers of last resort to those who could not afford to purchase care, and whose needs could not be met by the informal networks of family and neighbourhood; the post-WWII expansion of the social state created the financial conditions for an expansion of the voluntary sector both in partnership with, and independently of, government; an initial phase of retrenchment in the 1970s led to government contracting out of social-service delivery and a substantial role for the voluntary sector; a second phase of retrenchment beginning in the 1990s witnessed the growing transformation of non-profit organizations into mere agents of the state, and their consequent loss of independence and identity. She concludes that, while "the state is paying more, *what* is paid for has narrowed." She also points to the medicalization of home care, as "health care needs and services have trumped social care." Finally, she notes that the "emergence of the competitive, managerial state, wedded to a competitive contract culture, has also facilitated a massive re-allocation of state resources from non-profit voluntary organizations to for-profit organizations."

Tamara Daly's chapter is followed by three chapters that take different looks at the impact of home-care reform on home-care workers. In Chapter Three, Allison Williams looks back at the impact of the initial wave of labour-process restructuring on home care workers in the early to mid-nineties. Emphasizing the significance of public-sector employment and services for the advancement of women, Allison Williams also highlights the importance of occupational and geographical segmentation in shaping gender relations. Noting that "[o]ccupational segregation begins at home, as women's labour-market positions are linked to their household responsibilities," she points both to the ways in which "sex-role stereotyping (...) places women in jobs that are extensions of their personal lives," and public-sector cuts transfer work from waged to unwaged workers. She then presents the results of an in-depth study of the impact of restructuring on home-care workers in Northern Ontario, showing that nurses experienced deteriorating working conditions and greater stress on the job, because they were dissatisfied with their working time, because their control over their work diminished, and because their responsibilities increased.

Chapter Four picks up the story with the 1996 Conservative reform of home care, as Denise O'Connor analyzes the devastation wreaked upon agencies and their employees by the introduction of managed competition. She shows that the purchaser-provider split provided a mechanism for enforcing rationing of home care, while the creation of the CCACs enabled the provincial government to distance itself politically from the process of retrenchment it had set in motion. She then argues that the rigidities of the system have not only harmed the interests of provider agencies and workers, but led to a loss of efficiency and capacity in the home-care sector as a whole, notably in the form of worker flight to other occupations. Agencies are caught in a bind, because they face constantly rising costs, but are locked into contracts that fix prices over an extended period of time. They must look after people with increasingly complex needs, yet "are not compensated for ensuring their workers have continuous education." Workers face constant uncertainty, as their hourly wages are low, their working hours can fluctuate week to week, and there is little prospect for improvement, given the very tight circumstances faced by their employers.

Finally, Paul Leduc Browne's concluding chapter argues that managed competition exacerbates the effects of power structures already embedded in the division of home care labour, intensifying the clash between values intrinsic to the care relationship and the very different values imported into the care process by bureaucratic rationalization and commodification. Browne stresses the collective, reciprocal nature of care and its nature as a public good. He argues that the "logic of care suggests the need for a holistic approach at odds with the fragmentation and quantification of the labour process" brought about by bureaucratic and technocratic strategies to cut costs/raise profits in the public and private sectors. He rejects the market option in home-care reform and advocates a new model of social economy that would allow reciprocity to flourish within a context of state redistribution. He concludes by calling for "a form of accountability based on the democratic association of workers, users and their families," not just a top-down accountability based on cost-shifting.

Bibliography

Armstrong, Pat & Hugh Armstrong (1996). *Wasting Away: The Undermining of Canadian Health Care*, Toronto, Oxford University Press.

Brown, Lesley (ed.). *The New Shorter Oxford English Dictionary*, Vol. 1, Oxford, The Clarendon Press.

Browne, Paul Leduc (2000). *Unsafe Practices. Restructuring and Privatization in Ontario Health Care*, Ottawa, CCPA Books.

Browne, Paul Leduc (1999). *Our Growing Market Dependency and How to Reduce It*, Background Paper for the 1999 Alternative Federal Budget, Ottawa/Winnipeg, Canadian Centre for Policy Alternatives/CHO!CES, 1999.

Browne, Paul Leduc (1996). *Love in a Cold World? The Voluntary Sector in an Age of Cuts*, Ottawa, Canadian Centre for Policy Alternatives.

Browne, Paul Leduc & David Welch (2002). "In the Shadow of the Market: Ontario's Social Economy in the Age of Neo-Liberalism," in Yves Vaillancourt

& Louise Tremblay (eds.), *Social Economy: Health and Welfare in Four Canadian Provinces*, translated by Stuart Anthony Stilitz, Halifax, Fernwood Publishing, 101-134.

Caillé, Alain (2001). "La société mondiale qui vient," in Jean-Louis Laville et al., *Association, démocratie et société civile*, Paris, Éditions La Découverte et Syros.

Church, Elizabeth (1999). "Number of workers who care for elderly and children rising: study," *The Globe and Mail*, November 11th, B12.

Conference Board of Canada (1999). "Eldercare taking its toll on Canadian workers," news release, November 10th.

Enthoven, Alain C. (1993). "The History and Principles of Managed Competition," *Health Affairs*,12, 24-48.

Enthoven, Alain C. (1988). *Theory and Practice of Managed Competition in Health Care Finance*, Amsterdam, North-Holland.

Flynn, Rob, Gareth Williams & Susan Pickard (1996). *Markets and Networks: Contracting in Community Health Services*, Buckingham, Open University Press.

Foucault, Michel (1975). *Surveiller et punir. Naissance de la prison*, Paris, Gallimard.

Fuller, Colleen (2001). *Home Care: What We Have, What We Need*, Ottawa, Canadian Health Coalition.

Gagnon, Éric & Francine Saillant (2000). *De la dépendance et de l'accompagnement. Soins à domicile et liens sociaux*, with Catherine Montgomery, Steve Paquet & Robert Sévigny, Sainte-Foy, L'Harmattan/Presses de l'Université Laval.

Godbout, Jacques (2000). *Le don, la dette et l'identité. Homo donator vs homo oeconomicus*, Montréal, Boréal.

Gratzer, David (1999). *Code Blue: Reviving Canada's Health Care System*, Toronto, ECW Press.

Laville, Jean-Louis (ed.) (1994). *L'économie solidaire. Une perspectives internationale*, Paris, Desclée de Brouwer.

Laville, Jean-Louis & Marthe Nyssens (eds.) (2001). *Les services sociaux entre associations, État et marché. L'aide aux personnes âgées*, Paris, Éditions La Découverte et Syros.

Leys, Colin (2001). *Market-Driven Politics: Neoliberal Democracy and the Public Interest*, London, Verso.

Light, Donald W. (2001). "Health Care Markets: Theory and Practice," *International Encyclopedia of the Social and Behavioral Sciences*, Amsterdam, Elsevier Sciences Ltd.

Light, Donald W. (2000). "The Sociological Character of Health-Care Markets," in G.L. Albrecht, R. Fitzpatrick & S.C. Scrimshaw (eds.), *The Handbook of Social Studies in Health and Medicine*, London, Sage, 394-408.

Light, Donald W. (1995). "Homo Economicus: Escaping the traps of managed competition," *European Journal of Public Health*, 5,145-154.

Light, Donald W. (1994). "Comparative Models of 'Health Care' Systems," in P. Conrad & R. Kern (eds.), *The Sociology of Health and Illness*, New York, St. Martin's Press, 455-470.

Light, Donald W. (1993). "Escaping the traps of postwar Western medicine: how to maximize health and minimize expenses," *European Journal of Public Health*, 3, 281-289.

Marks, Lynne (1995). "Indigent Committees and Ladies' Benevolent Societies: Intersections of Public and Private Poor Relief in Late Nineteenth-Century Small-Town Ontario," *Studies in Political Economy*, 47.

Martin, Brendan (1993). *In the Public Interest? Privatization and Public Sector Reform*, London, Zed Books.

Maurutto, Paula (2003). *Governing Charities. Church and State in Toronto's Catholic Archdiocese, 1850-1950*, Montreal-Kingston, McGill-Queen's University Press.

O'Connor, James (1973). *The Fiscal Crisis of the State*, New York, St. Martin's Press.

Romanow, Roy (2002). *Building on Values: The Future of Health Care in Canada*, Final Report of the Commission on the Future of Health Care in Canada, November.

Saint-Martin, Denis (2001). "Les cabinets de conseil et la 're-marchandisation' de la politique sociale dans les États-providences de type libéral," *Lien social et Politiques—RIAC*, 45 (Spring), 131-144.

Scott, Katherine (2003). *Funding Matters: The Impact of Canada's New Funding Regime on Nonprofit and Voluntary Organizations*, Ottawa, Canadian Council on Social Development in collaboration with the Coalition of National Voluntary Organizations.

Serré, Marina & Frédéric Pierru (2001). "Les organisations internationales et la production d'un sens commun réformateur de la politique de protection maladie," *Lien social et Politiques—RIAC*, 45 (Spring), 109-128.

Shortt, S.E.D. (2001). *Borrowing Policy Misadventures from Abroad: Howe Not to Reform Canada's Health System*, Policy Working Paper 01-01, Kingston, Ontario, Queen's University Centre for Health Services and Policy Research.

Starr, Paul (1990). "The New Life of the Liberal State: Privatization and the Restructuring of State-Society Relations," in John Waterbury and Ezra Suleiman (eds.), *Public Enterprise and Privatization*, Boulder, Westview Press.

Starr, Paul (1988). "The Meaning of Privatization," *Yale Law and Policy Review*, 6, 6-41.

Twigg, Julia (2000a). "Carework as a Form of Bodywork," *Ageing and Society*, 20, 389-411.

Twigg, Julia (2000b). *Bathing—The Body and Community Care*, London, Routledge.

Valverde, Mariana (1995). "The Mixed Social Economy as a Canadian Tradition," *Studies in Political Economy*, 47.

Woolhandler S. & D.U. Himmelstein (1993). *Managed competition: a grimm fairytale*, Cambridge, Mass., Center for National Health Program Studies.

Wuthnow, Robert (1991). *Acts of Compassion: Caring for Others and Helping Ourselves*, Princeton, Princeton University Press.

Notes

[1] Community care access centres were originally established as formally autonomous non-profit corporations governed by boards representative of their communities. Although board members were initially appointed by the provincial government, many boards established procedures for ensuring their own renewal through election or co-optation. This came to an end in December 2001, when provincial legislation transformed community care access centres into statutory agencies with boards appointed by the Ontario government.

[2] An expression typically used by volunteers to explain why they have chosen to give of their time and labour to others.

[3] Most caregivers are women (see Armstrong and Kits in this volume). However, care is no more a special characteristic of women's nature, than it is a "product" to be delivered. To essentialize it in that way is to believe that some people (women) are good caregivers simply on the basis of who they are, rather than to understand that caring is complex, skilled labour that workers must learn to accomplish. This is not to deny that women's socialization may involve the acquisition of skills that are conducive to caregiving: "While not all emotional labour is carried out by women, it builds on skills women learn as part of what Oakley refers to as their 'long apprenticeship.'"(James, 1989, 37)

Similarly, emphasizing the dimension of giving and reciprocity in caregiving does not mean regarding it as some form of saintly altruism. Self-interest is not absent from giving (Godbout, 2000; Wuthnow, 1991), nor is power (physical, emotional, financial, professional), which can corrupt and undermine the relations of care (Gagnon & Saillant, 2000; Browne in this volume).

[4] In constant 2000 dollars.

[5] Since the great majority of people are forced to work for a wage for most of their lives, have limited time for family responsibilities, and often must migrate in search of employment, informal networks of care are often precarious and ephemeral, if they exist at all. Most wage earners are unable to pay for assistance and care. Wage earners (mostly women) are compelled to perform extraordinary amounts of carework parallel to their waged work or during their retirement, very much on their own, with very little outside support.

[6] In 1999-2000, Ontario's registered nurses working in home care made $16 to $23 an hour, while their counterparts in hospitals earned $19 to $28 an hour. Personal support workers made $5 to $8 an hour less in the community sector than in long-term-care facilities. (Browne, 2000)

7   "Privatization is a process whereby *activities, assets, costs, or control are shifted from the public to the for-profit private sector.* (...) the privatization of public services occurs when governments: cease altogether from paying for a service or providing it; still pay for a service, but no longer deliver it themselves, or do so less, instead turning to the private for-profit sector to do so; still provide the service, but require someone else, such as the user, to assume part or all of the cost; still provide and pay for a service, but manage and deliver it along the lines of a commercial, for-profit enterprise. Some of the key policies and policy instruments associated with privatization are service reductions, contracting out, public-private partnerships, cost shifting (user fees, delisting, de-insuring), commercialization, and organizational restructuring." (Browne, 2000, 2-3) In the field of Canadian health care, scarcely anyone advocates the complete abandonment of any state role. Some of those who argue for a greater role for the private sector in Canada's public health care system on the grounds of the supposed efficiency and capacity for innovation generated by markets and the profit motive, also accept that the state must play a role in ensuring equitable access to care and in controlling costs. Even the Fraser Institute, which unequivocally asserts the complete superiority of the private over the public sector in the production of goods and services, allows that the state should have a role in funding *medical savings accounts* upon which individual citizens would draw to pay for medical services. (Gratzer, 1999) For a critique of this idea, see Shortt (2001).

8   "[C]'est moins un modèle d'organisation précis et omnibus des systèmes de santé qu'un ensemble de principes d'action et d'outils que proposent ces organisations. Le répertoire néolibéral des organisations internationales repose ainsi à la fois sur un diagnostic (la crise d'efficience des sytèmes), un mot d'ordre (la concurrence encadrée) et des recettes inspirées du nouveau management public et de la 'gestion des soins'." (Serré & Pierru, 2001)

Chapter 1
Caregiving in Historical Perspective[1]
Pat Armstrong and Olga Kits

1. Introduction

Caregiving is not a simple act but rather a complex social relationship embedded in personal histories and located within specific conditions. These relationships can be found throughout our society and in a multitude of forms. Caregiving exists within health-care institutions and in hostels, in households and on the street. Where it happens, and with whom, changes over time and with place, even for the same individuals. Partners and friends, mothers and fathers, daughters and sons, relatives and strangers, old and young participate in caregiving, although there are clear patterns linked to gender, age, and social circumstance.

Most care is unpaid, done with little formal training and based on an existing relationship. Yet even the distinction between formal and informal care is far from simple. Some relatives are paid for such informal care; some begin as strangers; many have become quite skilled at caregiving and share the job with those who are part of the formal system.

To help sort through this complexity, the paper begins with a discussion of the diversity in caregiving relationships. It then moves on to consider what changed and did not change significantly in these relationships throughout the twentieth century. On the basis of this exploration of history and diversity, the final sections set out a framework for assessing legislation, regulations and policy that influence caregiving among adults.

2. Recognizing Caregiving in All its Diversity

2.1. What Is Involved in Caregiving?

The forms of care can be thought of as falling into four broad, overlapping categories. The most pervasive form is the management of care. (Rosenthal & Martin-Matthews, 1999) Almost all caregivers are involved in care management, but some caregivers are primarily managers. They find out about, and arrange for, formal services as well as ensure that the formal services are received. They act as case managers, determining hours of service and eligibility, making appointments and convincing care recipients to participate. They mediate between care recipients and paid care providers, and advocate on behalf of recipients for care inside or outside the home. This organization of care not only involves negotiation among paid providers and with the care recipient; it also involves negotiations among informal providers. Managing money, providing financial assistance, completing forms, assembling documents and organizing test results are all part of care management. Equally important, care management usually requires decision-making, often without the active participation of the person needing care. Each aspect of organizing care may involve conflicts; conflicts among formal and informal providers, conflicts between the groups and conflicts among any of the providers and the care recipient. This organization also requires cooperation among all of these participants and needs to be done even for people living in institutional settings. The need for such "orchestration of care," bureaucratic management and financial assistance (Rosenthal & Martin-Matthews, 1999, 17) varies over time, with illness and in relation to the availability of public support and services.

Another common form of caregiving involves what are in the literature on caregiving called *Instrumental Activities of Daily Living* (IADL). When people become ill, have day surgery, are released early from hospital, have more long-term disabilities or simply become frailer with old age, they require assistance with cooking, shopping, cleaning, laundry, and home maintenance tasks. They may also need help getting around, within and outside the house. People may require assistance with only some of these tasks, or with all of them. Residential care reduces the need for most, but not all, of this support.

Some people require more than assistance with figuring out which services to use or with daily survival in their homes. They need direct help with much more personal and more medical aspects of care. This third form of care is referred to as assistance with the Activities of

Daily Living (ADL), and includes dressing, bathing, eating, using the toilet, brushing their teeth and combing their hair. It also includes taking medications, inserting needles and using a variety of equipment such as catheters, oxygen masks and feeding tubes. Here, too, residential care fills much of the need but still must be supplemented by informal caregivers in many cases.

Finally, there is the form of care that should pervade all the others but may also exist on its own. Everyone requires social and emotional support. But those who have undergone surgery, live with disabilities or live into frail old age have particular needs for companionship, for touch, for listeners and talkers and for comfort of all sorts, especially if they are not able to leave their home or institution. The need is particularly great in the case of palliative care. Caregivers may be engaged in only one of these forms, but many provide all four forms of care.

2.2. What Care is Provided?

What care is provided depends on a range, and mix, of factors. Government policies play a critical role in what care is provided, especially in terms of formal services. The *Canada Health Act* requires that all medically necessary care provided by a doctor or hospital be offered to Canadian residents without charge and in an accessible manner. As care moves outside these boundaries, however, there is no national standard for formal, public care. This is why the National Forum on Health, a group appointed by Prime Minister Chrétien to advise on health policy, recommended national homecare and pharmacare programs in its 1997 report. (National Forum on Health, 1997) The Forum had little to say about long-term care facilities, although they too are largely outside the *Canada Health Act*.

In terms of homecare, provinces provide professional services such as nursing and physiotherapy without charge but many provinces charge user fees for homemaking, personal care, housecleaning or transportation. Some provide supplies and equipment without cost while others charge; some cover required medications while others do not. Some have extensive provisions for respite care, while others provide very limited access. There is also considerable variation in eligibility rules and in the limits placed on services, creating even greater differences in supports available. (Morris et al., 1999; CHCA, 1998)

Access to institutional facilities also differs somewhat across provinces. While only 1 percent of Canadians live in such facilities (Trottier et al, 2000, 49), the eligibility requirements, the location, the number of beds available, the nature of the services provided and the fees charged vary in ways that limit options for those care givers and care recipients who need such services.

Government policies on direct and indirect financial support also influence the care provided. Direct financial support for care providers is quite limited and equally varied. For the decade between 1984 and 1994, Nova Scotia provided compensation to caregivers, most of whom were young females in rural areas. This means-tested program paid considerably less than minimum wage for quite heavy workloads, and primarily served to reinforce caregiving as undervalued women's work. (Keefe & Fancey, 1997) Québec now provides up to $600 to caregivers to purchase respite care, again based on a means-tested system. Most provincial financial support, however, comes indirectly through the tax system for deductions related to medical expenses, attendant allowances, and disability. Since 1998, the Federal Government has offered the Caregiver Tax Credit. This allows those who live with, and care for an elderly relative to claim up to $400, if the claimant's annual income is less than $13,853. (Jenson & Jacobzone, 2000, 26) These deductions and credits mean little to the many low income women who provide care, given that they have little income from which to deduct the taxes and that they may have "to absorb the cost of additional caregiving services before being eligible for reimbursements." (Keefe & Fancey, 1997, 256) There is, however, little research on the impact of direct financial compensation programmes on care givers or recipients. (Keefe & Fancey, 1997, 275)

Access to formal services and other government financial supports for caregivers are clearly important to both care providers and care recipients. Yet, contrary to much popular discussion, the availability of care does not automatically mean less informal care is provided. Indeed, study after study demonstrates that between 85 percent and 90 percent of care is provided informally. (Denton, 1997; Ontario,

1991, 210; Connidis, 1983) Even these figures may understate the amount of informal care provided, given that "it is probably also the case that a lot more help is exchanged in families than is ever reported in surveys because people do not consciously think about what they are doing in providing help." (Rosenthal & Stone, 1999, 9) This is particularly the case for women who may see their caregiving work as a simple extension of usual practices. As a variety of researchers explain, for women, caring about someone very often is equated with caring for them and the work as well as the skill of care becomes invisible in the process. (Dalley, 1988; Neysmith, 2000; Finch & Groves, 1983)

Informal and formal care are complementary rather than alternative forms of support. (Penning, 2000; Rosenthal & Martin-Matthews, 1999; Keefe & Fancey, 1997; Chappell & Blandford, 1991) Instead of replacing informal caregivers, formal services are more likely to fill in when there are no informal caregivers or to provide some services that are supplemental to informal care. (Denton, 1997, 30) As a study conducted for Statistics Canada concludes, "the informal network operates in concert with the formal delivery system" (Wilkins & Beaudet, 2000, 45) and the availability of formal services does not mean families and friends shirk their responsibilities. Nor does access to formal services mean people rush to use them. The overwhelming majority of health problems are managed through self-care. And "most people who consult a physician have tried treating themselves before seeking medical advice." (Morrongiello & Gottlieb, 2000, 38-39) This is especially the case for women.

In addition to providing formal services, governments also influence the care provided through employment regulations. No jurisdiction requires employers to provide "caregiver leave." However some employment or labour standards legislation allows short-term and unpaid leave. (Canada, 1996) While most collective agreements simply reflect the statutory emphasis on parental, sick and bereavement leave, some include additional leave provisions for those with disabilities and for personal reasons. The Public Service Alliance of Canada, for example, has negotiated leave with pay for family related responsibilities. In this case, family is broadly defined to include not only spouses and common-law partners but also any of the children dependent on them. Parents as well as stepparents or foster parents are considered family and so are any relatives permanently residing in the employee's household or with whom the employee resides. The paid leave is only for a maximum of five days, although leave without pay is allowed for long-term care of a parent for up to five years. (Canada, 2000)

Physical location also influences what care is provided, in part because formal services vary within provinces. Urban populations often have better access to care supports than do rural ones. "Poor quality housing and insufficient health and social services characterize many rural communities. Distance makes access to services more difficult and adversely affects rural women's ability to provide care." (Blakley & Jaffe, 1999, 3) Declining employment opportunities in rural areas, combined with health care reforms, mean fewer resources for increasing needs. This, in turn, means greater inequality in coping ability. (Cloutier-Fisher & Joseph, 2000, 1083) Native communities in particular frequently lack formal, community-based services. (Buchignani & Armstrong-Esther, 1999)

Similarly, those living in large urban centers are more likely to find services that respond to their particular cultural or religious practices. For example, concentrated populations mean urban Japanese Canadians can access some culturally sensitive programs. Such access can affect whether or not they use formal services at all, regardless of need, and may matter as much as quality and location in seeking care. (Chubachi, 1999, 1)

Physical location also matters in terms of informal caregiving. The further away friends, relatives and volunteers are, the more difficult it is to provide direct personal care. Children move away for education or employment; people immigrate, leaving their relatives behind. Nevertheless, many people do provide care-at-a-distance, especially care that is of the management sort. (Rosenthal & Martin-Matthews, 1999) Or they move themselves or others in order to give care. In 1996, nearly half a million Canadians moved to give or receive care. The majority of those who moved were married, more than a third had children under the age of fifteen and had paid work. Those who move, then, have a range of caregiving responsibilities. While daughters are the most likely to make such moves, a significant proportion are friends (18 percent) or other relatives. (Cranswick, 1999, 11-12) Living arrangements do not play a central role in emotional support, and may be provided in person, by telephone, e-mail or letter from anywhere. But living with someone may be the major determinant of help with activities of daily living; even more important than a marital or blood relationship. (Chappell & Blandford, 1991)

Social location matters at least as much as physical location in terms of what care is provided. Being a mother, a daughter or a spouse is critical, because daughters and mothers are the most common primary caregivers, followed by spouses, friends and volunteers. (Campbell & Martin-Matthews, 2000; Frederick & Fast, 1999; Morris et al., 1999) We have little Canadian information on caregiving among same-sex couples or singles, but we do know that the gay and lesbian communities have formed support organizations and care services, especially for those suffering from HIV/AIDS. (Taylor, forthcoming)

Gender and income also have a profound influence on what care is provided. According to a recent study, "Women family members were expected to supplement home-care services without pay and at great personal expense in terms of their own health, incomes, benefits, career development and pension accumulation, while men were not under as much pressure to do so." (Morris et al., 1999, vi) Financial costs were picked up by recipients and families; those without money do without and those who were poor or isolated fare worst of all. De-institutionalization, early discharge, day surgery and cutbacks in public health services all shift more care work and care costs onto individuals and families, and especially onto women. The more care is privatized, the more the poor cannot afford care. Those without homes or relatives are particularly at risk of not receiving care. (Bernier & Dallaire, 2000; Wilson & Howard, 2000; Armstrong & Armstrong, 1999; Fuller, 1999; Gurevich, 1999)

Finally, the needs of the person receiving care are a critical component in what care is provided. Those who are expected to recover after day surgery or early discharge from a hospital place high, immediate demands on caregivers for assistance in the full range of caregiving activities. Patients recovering from cardiac surgery, for example, require monitoring for their heart rate, for infection and for wound healing; they need reassurance and comfort, as well as help in eating, bathing, going to the toilet, keeping the house in order and in managing their diet and exercise program. (King & Koop, 1999) However, these demands are expected to diminish over time until eventually care is no longer required. The situation is quite different for someone suffering from Alzheimer's or Multiple Sclerosis. Care needs can only increase with time and last until death.

Care varies as well with the stage of an illness. Initially cancer care may mainly involve management and emotional support. During and after treatment it may require the full range of care forms. If the cancer is successfully treated, the need for all but emotional and social support may disappear. But if the treatment fails, then care needs gradually, or perhaps quite quickly, increase, ending over a relatively short term in death.

Chronic diseases too have stages that create varying needs for care. Multiple Sclerosis, for instance, may go into remission, allowing a person to live relatively independently for long periods. Arthritis and rheumatism may mean that only heavy housework and house maintenance are a problem for a long time, with more needs appearing over time. Stroke patients may fully recover after temporary severe disability, or become quite dependent for the rest of their lives. (Stewart, 2000)

Some chronic diseases and disabilities, however, exist from birth and mean that life is only possible with the provision of the full range of care, or with one form of care throughout life. (The Roeher Institute, 2001) Others may become paraplegic suddenly as a result of an accident. Care throughout life, or for most of it, is not uncommon. Of the 53 women interviewed for a study of rural caregivers, 5 had been caregiving for more than 20 years and one had been doing so for 35 years. Such caregivers provide care "all the time," often with little support from the formal system. (Blakley & Jaffe, 1999, 5)

In short, what unpaid care is provided depends on government policies and on the health issue, as well as on physical and social location. Formal care does not substitute for informal care. Rather, most care is informal or self-care and formal services supplement them.

2.3. Who Needs Care?

The short answer to the question, "who needs care?" is "everyone at some time in their lives." The surprising answer is not necessarily seniors. According to a recent study based on Statistics Canada data, "when it comes to receiving assistance from others, similar proportions of seniors and non-seniors received assistance. And across age groups, only a minority reported that they received no assistance." (Keating, Fast & Frederick, 1999, 17) Another Statistics Canada report describes seniors as a diverse group that is aging well. (Lindsay, 1999) More than nine out of ten seniors live in a private household, and although over half say they get some help with household chores and personal tasks, half also say that they provide care to others. (Lindsay, 1999, 25; Robb et al., 1999) In other words, care is for many seniors an exchange of services. Nevertheless, a significant number of seniors do need care. Of the 30 percent who required health-related personal assistance, three out of four needed assistance with daily living activities and a quarter required extensive personal care. Women were not only more likely to need care but also more likely to have those needs go unmet. The lower the income and education, the greater the unmet need. And living alone also meant that the necessary care was less likely to be provided. (Chen & Wilkins, 1998) While most of this care is provided by informal caregivers, losing a partner is a major factor in entry into the use of formal home-care services. (Wilkins & Beaudet, 2000, 39)

The number of people with long-term disabilities is also growing. Like seniors, they are a diverse group. Their disabilities may be physical, mental or intellectual, or a combination of these. These disabilities may be life long, result from a particular event or develop with age. The disability may mean only one form of care is required or it may mean the entire array of supports is necessary, during one period or throughout life. (The Roeher Institute, 2001) Take those with an intellectual disability, for example. Better care and better conditions for health mean that only now are many people with intellectual disabilities living to grow old. Many were placed in institutions, but in recent years have moved into communities where they may no longer have family connections, or their families feel hesitation about taking on their care and guilt about placing them in an institution. (Salvatori et al., 1998)

Shorter term, but often more intense care is required by those with terminal illnesses and by those released early from hospital or undergoing day surgery. The increased demand for care after early release from hospital or day surgery strains existing community resources, often leaving the frail elderly who have been receiving care without much formal assistance. (Cloutier-Fisher & Joseph, 2000) Palliative care services are beginning to appear both as formal residential services and as support for informal caregivers in the home.

2.4. Who Provides Care?

The clear answer to the "Who provides" question is women. As daughters, mothers, partners, friends, or as volunteers, women are the overwhelming majority of unpaid primary caregivers and spend more time than men in providing care. Women are much more likely than men to do personal care and offer emotional support. Men's contributions are more likely to be concentrated in care management or household maintenance, shopping or transportation. (Campbell & Martin-Matthews, 2000; Rosenthal & Martin-Matthews, 1999) In other words, women are more likely to provide the care that is daily and inflexible while men provide care that can be more easily planned and organized around paid work. (Gignac, Kelloway & Gottlieb, 1996) And men are more likely than women to get formal help when they do provide care, on the assumptions that they must have paid jobs and that they lack the skills necessary to provide care. (King & Koop, 1999; Morris et al., 1999; Aronson & Neysmith, 1997; Keefe & Fancey, 1997) Yet women provide personal care even when they have paid jobs, although higher income women may be able to become more care managers than care providers. (Rosenthal & Martin-Matthews, 1999, 7) The little research that has been done about differences among women caregivers suggests that income and education matter at least as much as culture in terms of the kinds and amounts of care provided. (Chubachi, 1999; Dorazio-Migliore, 1999) While most women want to provide various kinds of informal care, they do not want to be "conscripted" into this relationship. (National Forum of Health, 1997, 19) And the poorer women are, regardless of their culture, the more likely they are to have little choice about providing care. (Morris et al., 1999)

Some men have provided, and continue to provide, the full range of care forms. Like women, they care for their spouses. However, fewer men are called on for such care because their wives usually outlive them, given women's greater longevity and the pattern of men marrying women significantly younger than themselves. Men care for their parents too, providing up to a quarter of the care. (Campbell & Martin-Matthews, 2000) Men also care for their same sex partners, and serve as volunteers who manage care, provide transport and support, deliver meals and do household chores. (Taylor, forthcoming; Campbell & Martin-Matthews, 2000; McCann & Wadsworth, 1992) And like women, men may provide care to siblings, in-laws or other relatives. (Buchignani & Armstrong-Esther, 1999)

Friends also provide considerable caregiving, although we know less about them than we do about the spouses, mothers and children who are caregivers. A Statistics Canada study found that nearly one in five of those who had moved in order to provide care were friends, rather than relatives, suggesting that friends do much more than offer the occasional visit. (Cranswick, 1999, 12)

We know even less about differences among caregivers related to culture. The research that does exist does not indicate major differences in the provision of care but some in the stated commitment to care. For example, Japanese Canadians express a high commitment to filial obligation. This is reflected in the provision of emotional support but not in support through financial or other services. (Kobayashi, 2000, 15) Some cultural groups are also much more likely than others to live in households that hold several generations, suggesting cross-generational caregiving. But this is not necessarily the case. While for example East Indian immigrants tend to live in multi-generational households, it is important not to assume that this, like the lower use of formal services, simply indicates cultural choices. This pattern may be as much about immigration regulations requiring support for sponsored relatives and limited economic resources as it is about preference. (Dhawan, 1998) That Chinese, Greek and Italian elderly are less likely to live alone than are other Canadians may reflect low incomes, lack of pensions and immigration rules as much as cultural values. (Brotman, 1998) Similarly, the fact that Native seniors are much more likely to live with relatives than are other Canadians may reflect poverty as much as choice or values. (Buchignani & Armstrong-Esther, 1999)

Like sponsored immigrants, spouses face rules governing support. The rules are fairly clear in terms of financial support, but less clear when it comes to providing direct care services. It is not evident that spousal support means you could take your partner to court to demand they change your diapers, insert your catheter or attach your oxygen mask. Certainly many of the policies and regulations in health care assume such support, especially from women, and enforce it through a failure to provide alternatives or through regulations. In Ontario, for example, government guidelines for in-home services say that people are not eligible for services until they have exhausted the support capacities of their family and friends and without regard to whether the caregivers are employed or not. (Armstrong & Armstrong, 1999, 22-23) Who constitutes a family for the purposes of providing such care, however, is not clear even in the regulations.

Children also can face legal obligations for support of their parents. These filial responsibility laws require children to provide support if parents need support, have supported the children in the past and if the children can afford to provide support. Sons are more likely, given higher work wages, to be able to afford financial assistance. It is perhaps not surprising that these laws are seldom used, in part, because many sons do support their parents when they can, just as spouses and same-sex couples and friends do. When they cannot or when they reject their responsibility, the enforcement of these filial laws can undermine family relationships.(Bracci, 2000; Snell, 1990)

Employees also have legal obligations; ones that may prevent rather than promote caregiving. (MacBride-King, 1999) One in four employees provide care, and a large proportion of care providers is employed. Not surprisingly, those with both eldercare and childcare responsibilities, most of whom are women, are the most likely to lose time at work as a result of caregiving. (Cranswick, 1999, Table 5) The very limited leave allowed for such care, combined with very few protections from being fired when caregiver stress leads to missed time at their paid jobs, mean that caregivers are very vulnerable at work. Those who care for people unrelated by blood or marriage may be particularly at risk.

3. Care and Consequences

Although caregiving and care receiving are about relationships, much of the research on the impact of caregiving has focused on the negative consequences for providers and viewed care recipients as objects rather than as participatory subjects. Not surprisingly, caregiver burden is a common theme in the literature.

There are many, and varied, aspects to this burden. Rural women who provide care describe feeling frustrated, especially with the repetitiveness of the tasks, and the problem of dealing with the frustration of the care recipient. (Blakley & Jaffe, 1999) They have to convince their husbands to allow them to bathe them and, like others who care for younger adults with severe physical disabilities, describe the "difficult and potentially hazardous situations resulting from a combination of the weight of the person being bathed and the lack of strength of both parties." (Gutman, 1995, 26) Lack of training for what is highly skilled caregiving also creates additional stress on relationships. For many caregivers, the most emotionally upsetting activities are those related to bladder and bowel management, in part because they are such intimate tasks. Male caregivers found bathing their wives disturbing for similar reasons. (Gutman, 1995, 26-27) Rural caregivers feel ineffective in dealing with mood swings of the care recipient and with their own guilt, guilt about being healthy, guilt about not understanding the illness and guilt about not making the right choices for the care recipient. (Blakley & Jaffe, 1999) Such guilt is widely shared among caregivers, especially by the women who provide most of the care. This guilt may be compounded by their role as sole confidante and decision-maker and by cultural pressures. (Dorazio-Migliore, 1999) Caregivers who move to provide care, like those who live-in or close-by, report changes in their sleep patterns, a decline in overall health, depression, a reduction in their social activities and holidays, and extra expenses. (Cranswick, 1999, 12) A study of caregivers for those with Parkinson's suggests that the strain is greater the closer the caregiver is to the recipient.(Moore, 1997, 66) In other words, loving the recipient may make it harder to care.

Stress of all sorts is a recurring theme, as is family conflict over who provides care and what kind of care is required. Conflicts may also arise between informal and formal caregivers, over what care should be provided and how it should be provided. Moreover, shifting care to homes means that formal services invade the household and "boundaries separating these domains" are continually crossed, creating greater strain on the entire household. (Ward-Griffin, 1998, ii) New policy initiatives urge partnerships between families and paid providers, but this may well be more an exploitative relationship than a partnership one, especially if the primary purpose is the reduction of public expenditure. In the partnership, "most family caregivers were left socially isolated without adequate resources to provide care. Intentionally or not, holding family caregivers accountable for the provision of care without adequate resources is completely unacceptable." (Ward-Griffin & McKeever, 2000, 101) Indeed, these researchers, on nurse/family relationships warn that "failure to provide resources to help family members provide care could risk even further increases in health costs, as injuries or illness"result for caregivers. Moreover, "failure to provide resources to help family members provide care could risk even further increases in health-care costs, as injuries or illnesses of the elder and/or family caregiver ensue." (Ward-Griffin & McKeever, 2000, 101) Privacy is reduced for the entire household and for their relationships. Even before the most recent cutbacks in services, research indicated that caregivers have higher rates of affective and anxiety disorders that noncaregivers and use mental health services twice as much. (Cochrane, Goering & Rogers, 1997, 1) Caregivers for people with dementia are particularly at risk, and among those, people whose first language is neither English nor French are especially fragile. (Meshefedjian et al., 1998) Immigrants may feel particularly isolated and limited in their access to services that meet their needs. This may contribute to depression, with those who have no outside help suffering the most.(Dhawan, 1998, 25)

Caregiving can mean career interruption, time lost from work, financial loss and, especially for women, even job loss. (Statistics Canada, 1997) Indeed, women feel much greater tension than men, between their caregiving and their paid work, and between their caregiving and other family responsibilities. This is not surprising, given that women do more of the personal care and domestic work. (Rosenthal & Martin-Matthews, 1999; Gignac, Kelloway & Gottlieb, 1996) For both women and men, the consequences of such interruptions can be felt far into the future in terms of low pensions and benefits in their own old age.

Although friends and volunteers provide considerable caregiving, virtually all of this caregiving burden research has been done on relatives, especially on the mothers, wives and daughters who do the majority of the care. This lack of research may not simply reflect a failure to recognize their contribution, however. It may also reflect the fact that friends and volunteers have more choice about where and when they provide care, as well as about what care they provide. There is also a lack of research on same-sex partners, but there is little reason to believe the burden would be lighter for them.

There is considerable discussion in the literature about the subjective factors, such as negative attitudes and cultural values towards caregiving that influence the impact on the caregiver. However, "a belief one is ill-equipped to meet the demands of caregiving may not be unrealistic. Economic factors, a lack of instrumental support or caregiver illness may greatly impede one's ability to cope and may thus be a realistic, objective perception." (O'Rourke et al., 1996) In other words, caregivers may perceive a burden because there is one. This is especially the case for those who must provide long-term and constant care. (The Roeher Institute, 2001; Echenberg, 1998)

It should be emphasized, however, that caregiving also has rewards. Caregivers experience warmth and satisfaction; they get joy from helping others and often feel rewarded through the personal interaction and the very real support they often receive in return. (MacBride-King, 1999) Yet, like most human relationships, caregivers' experiences are contradictory. (Aronson, 1998) Resentment, stress, frustration and ill health too often occur along with the good parts, and are most likely to occur in the absence of support, relief and choice. The strain is too often manifested as abuse (Spencer, Ashfield & Vanderbijl, 1996), not only of the elderly but also of the disabled whatever their age. Older people with intellectual disabilities may be doubly disadvantaged by prejudice against both the elderly and the disabled. Support groups, while often offered as an inexpensive way to relieve the burden of caregiving, have little impact, especially in the absence of other, more material supports. (Colantonio, Cohen & Corlett, 1998; Lavoie, 1995)

What about the burden on care recipients? We know less about this burden or about their views on the relationship. What we do know suggests they too have burdens in addition to those caused by their physical or mental problems or both, especially when their low incomes and cutbacks in services eliminate choices about care. Care receivers may be placed in a position of "compulsory acquiescence"; not primarily by their informal care providers but rather by the public system's failure to offer them choices. Elderly women experience conflicts between their need for support and the expectation of self-sufficiency, as well as between the media panic over the costs of an aging population and the system's failure to recognize the specificity of their individual needs. Seeking to maintain reciprocity and their pride, these women feel the strain of limiting their demands and the strain within their relationships. (Aronson, 1990, 244-245) Like caregivers, they experience guilt and frustration. (Aronson, 1998) On the other hand, having a partner can make a significant difference, even in ill health. Indeed, "married seniors in poor health enjoy a high level of emotional support and are just as socially engaged as those in good health." (Crompton & Kemeny, 1999, 26) It seems likely this is the case with couples or others who are not married but who have enjoyed a long life together. As is the case with caregivers, there appear to be significant differences in the burdens felt by women and men. "Female respondents described feeling guilty when their husbands did laundry and prepared meals if they had never been involved in these tasks before." At the same time, these women with osteoarthritis or osteoporosis defined help from spouses with mobility, at home or in the community, as simply part of the relationship. Men, on the other hand, did not usually see help from a spouse with such household tasks or with personal care as dependence. (Cott & Gignac, 1999)

In sum, caring is about complex relationships that take a wide variety of forms. These relationships are shaped not simply by individuals, their culture and their personal histories but also by the services, supports and alternatives available to them. The focus in recent research has been on the caregiver in part because the conditions for caregiving are changing significantly, and changing in ways that make caregiving more difficult and varied. "Those with more resources, by virtue of class, race or age, will be better able to offset the costs of caring, whether by purchasing private help or by being able to negotiate public resources from a more privileged position." (Aronson & Neysmith, 1997, 51) And those in stable relationships supported by adequate income and services are in the best position to give and receive care.

4. The Context of Caregiving: One Hundred Years

Context matters. The context shapes the possibilities for caregiving, setting the stage for patterns in care. Much of the discussion about caregiving, however, is based on myths about the past and present. Such myths often distort our assessment of legislative, regulatory and policy options, so it is important to look at what has changed and what has not changed much over the last hundred years.

4.1. What Has Not Changed Significantly Over the Last Hundred Years

Neither government fears that families will shirk their responsibilities for care nor fears of an aging population are new, although neither fear has much justification. One hundred years ago the majority of elderly lived in private households and were listed as family heads or spouses of family heads, indicating relative economic and social self-sufficiency. (Montigny & Chambers, 1998, 460) This is still the case today, with most of the aged living with spouses and only a minority listed as dependent on others. Over 90 percent of seniors now live in a private household, most with their immediate family. (Lindsay, 1999, 24) At the same time, living in extended families is not uncommon today. Indeed, the number of three-generation households increased in the last decade of the twentieth century, with half of them headed by immigrants and 40 percent including someone with some disability. (Che-Alford & Hamm, 1999)

Like today, many adult children continued to live with their parents because they could not find paid work that would support them in living independent lives. (Dillon, 1998) It was in rural areas that the old were most likely to live with their children while overcrowding and poverty in urban areas made co-residency much less likely. (Struthers, 1994, 52-53) Although this co-residence may well mean that adult children are providing some care for their elderly parents, it also often means they themselves receive support. In both periods, women without spouses were more likely than men to live with their children because they did not have enough income to live on their own. Such women were likely to be contributing members of the household, especially in rural areas, and not simply dependent care recipients. (Montigny, 1997)

Even though the elderly were and are mainly self-sufficient, concern about the costs of an aging population are recurring themes throughout the century. The end of the nineteenth century, like the end of the twentieth, saw the "rapid increase in demand for institutional accommodation for the province's aged population during a period of fiscal restraint" (Davies, forthcoming; Montigny, 2000), while governments blamed families for shirking responsibilities. A century ago, 3 percent of the elderly and of those with disabilities lived in institutions while about 1 percent does so today. (Montigny, 1997)

The government response then, like today, was to restrict admission to institutions and argue that care was a family obligation. Then, like now, some families were not able or willing to provide support and providing support often caused conflicts within families. The recognition of such conflicts can be found historically in the "elaborate provisions in wills and maintenance agreements" obliging support.

(Bruce Elliott in Dillon, forthcoming) Similarly, filial laws first introduced in Quebec in 1866 indicate that children did not always support their parents in their old age, although the limited cases of actual enforcement of these laws suggest either that most children provided support or that parents were unwilling to force the case. (Snell, 1990; Guest, 1980) Governments also began, as early as 1906, to discuss pensions for the elderly and other forms of support for the disabled, because many of the elderly and disabled did not have families providing care. (Guest, 1980)

Although there is considerable evidence that support for those needing care has long been recognized as a collective and public responsibility (Davies, forthcoming; McDaniel & Lewis, 1998), there is even stronger evidence indicating state commitment to and enforcement of family responsibility. (Snell, 1996) Yet in both periods, there is little evidence to support the claim that many families abandon their responsibilities for the elderly and the younger disabled or that age alone creates dependency. Most families then and now care for their kin. Marriage vows once involved spouses promising to love, honour and obey in sickness and in health, and this is still the expectation today whether or not such vows are involved. Equally important, concerns about an aging population are not new and such concerns persist even in the face of evidence indicating that the overwhelming majority of the elderly do not rely on the state for care. Indeed, many of the elderly themselves provide care in ways that relieve the state of care costs.

Charities and volunteers have not abandoned their responsibilities during the twentieth century either. At the end of the nineteenth century, governments like the one in Ontario "came to accept a great deal of responsibility for the care of the ill, the insane, the destitute, and the dependent aged." (Montigny, 2000, 74) At the same time, much of this care was provided through the funding of charitable or lay organizations. This is still the case today. Canadians also continue to volunteer in large numbers, through both formal and informal networks to deliver food and to transport people to care services, to provide information, to visit, to offer personal support and care. (Statistics Canada, 1998; Chappell & Prince, 1997) "One-fifth of caregivers were neighbours and friends, evidence that the caring society also reaches beyond family obligations." (Keating, Fast & Frederick, 1999, 53) Moreover, volunteers are now doing a considerable amount of caregiving that would otherwise be done by paid workers, "transformed into wageless workers with less control over their caring work." (Esteves, 2000, 154)

The notion that families and charities provided all the care desired, and did so well, is often linked to the notion of everyone living in large, rural households based on a heterosexual couple still with the same partner they married in their teens. Yet households were much more diverse than that. Women and men often waited until they had the economic resources to marry and a significant number never married at all. Death from childbirth, from injury, from infectious diseases and other illnesses meant that many heterosexual couples found themselves widowed early. Remarriage, and along with it the blending of households, was common. While the law made divorce difficult to get, desertion was not uncommon and there is every reason to believe that the deserters and deserted later took up residence with others, usually without the benefit of marriage. Nor was it unknown for friends to live together. What is unknown is how many of these friends were also sexual partners. Urban households, especially those that were not affluent, tended to be quite small. (Parr, 1995) Urban households were also much more likely to contain recent immigrants who usually occupied areas of the city recently abandoned by other immigrants only to be replaced themselves by the next wave of immigration. (Porter, 1965) In some areas, such as British Columbia, there were far more men than women and the men often looked after and lived with each other. (Davies, forthcoming) In other areas, like Paris Ontario, women formed the primary labour force and provided important support networks for each other. (Davies, forthcoming; Eichler, 2000; Smart, 2000; Bradbury, 1993; Parr, 1990)

Nor can it be assumed that all families were based on a mother at home, with time to care for others while father earned the bread needed by the entire household. In rural areas, most women worked hard in production on the farm and had little spare time for caregiving. In urban areas, many men did not earn enough to support the family

The Commodity of Care 43

and the entire household entered the labour force. For those who were not married, paid work was often the only option. However, that paid work frequently involved providing care in someone else's home. In fact, the household with a male breadwinner earning enough income to support the family and with a woman who had enough time to provide care was a dominant family form only for a brief period following the Second World War. It was a form made possible both by high, secure and well-paid male employment and by a welfare state that offered not only considerable support but also a redistribution of economic resources. (Bradbury, 1993; Cohen, 1988)

4.2. What has Changed Significantly over the Last Hundred Years?

While there are very similar patterns in some areas over the last century, there are also some quite radical differences that create different conditions and demands for care. One of the most obvious changes is health. Better nutrition, transportation, working and housing conditions, along with more formal education, have all contributed to better health. At the beginning of the twentieth century, Canadians were not generally in good health and even the Sickness Survey of 1950-51 showed that "Canadians were not a healthy people." (Taylor, 1978, 5) Relatively secure employment and decent wages for many men and some women made an important difference to the health not only of the men but also of those who were largely dependent on them. So did the welfare state. Much of the planning in the aftermath of World War Two was based on the assumption that "organized provision will be made in the post-war world for the risks and contingencies of family life that are beyond the capacity of most of them to finance adequately from their own resources." (Marsh, 1975, 7)

Under the welfare state, income tax was changed to make those with higher incomes pay a greater share. This progressive taxation strategy contributed to redistribution of resources. Labour standards legislation and worker's compensation protected many workers, as did unemployment insurance, maternity leave and both public and private job-related pension schemes. Unionization became easier and more effective in gaining rights for workers. Human Rights legislation supported equity in a variety of situations and allowed affirmative action in others. The universal pension for elderly people reduced poverty and dependence in old age, while the Canada Assistance Plan, the means-tested Guaranteed Income Supplement linked to the Old Age Pension and various plans for those with disabilities all helped reduce inequality and improve health. (The Roeher Institute, 2001; Echenberg, 1998; McGilly, 1991; Banting, 1982; Guest, 1980) More public transport made more people mobile and public housing gave some a home. Innovations in housing strategies for the elderly and the disabled helped many live with dignity without depending on their families. (Doyle, 1989; Gutman, 1989; Gutman & Blackie, 1988; Blackie et al., 1985; CMHC, 1983) Universal public education from kindergarten to high school also contributed to greater equality and thus to health. (Myles, 2000; Banting, 1982; Guest, 1980) Unlike most of the support in the nineteenth century, many of these programs were defined as rights of citizenship rather than as charity schemes targeted at the deserving. (Armstrong, 1997)

Together, and combined with the move from primary resources and goods production to services and the accompanying urbanization, these welfare state measures contributed to a significant decline in the time men spent in the labour force. At the beginning of the century, men began paid work at an early age, worked long hours, had few or no vacations and stayed working until they were no longer physically able, often gradually reducing paid work and dying shortly after they finally quit. (Chappell, Strain & Blandford, 1986, 10) Now full-time paid employment cannot begin at least until age 16, and for most it begins far later, after years of formal education. And for many it ends at least at age 65, where compulsory retirement is legal, and pensions or early retirement packages mean some people leave even before then. Most men can then expect to live well beyond retirement from their paid work. This development may have contradictory effects on men, and the extent to which they enjoy being out of the labour force will depend in part on both what kind of job they leave and what kind of income they have.

Public health measures such as immunization, food inspection, drug regulation and water treatment reduced the spread of infectious and other diseases. Universal health care coverage for hospitals and doctors were part of this welfare state development, as were the expansion of residential care facilities and public home-care services. Universal coverage, combined with new developments in drugs and techniques, were major factors in falling infant and maternal mortality rates, as well as in the successful treatment of many illnesses. (Armstrong & Armstrong, 1998) By the 1990s, the overwhelming majority of Canadians rated their health as good to excellent—even among those over age 75—and Canada was near the top on most health indicators. (Rosenberg & Moore, 1997) Many more people survived with significant or severe disabilities and with chronic diseases. Those with intellectual disabilities, for example, are finally getting to live into old age. (Salvatori et al., 1998) Old age also became older, as longevity increased. Nearly 12 percent of the population was over 65 in 1999 and those over 85 are the fastest growing segment. Women are the overwhelming majority of the old old. (Ontario Human Rights Commission, 2000)

Of course, the welfare state was far from perfect and far from successful in eliminating inequality. Many more men than women were able to benefit from the employment-related programs and few with long-term disabilities had access to these rights-based schemes. (Echenberg, 1998) Welfare programs often served to reinforce dependency without alleviating poverty and offered support as charity. Nevertheless, contributions of the welfare state to reducing inequality have become increasingly clear as its demise coincides with growing inequality among both individuals and families. (Davies et al., 2001; Sauvé, 1999; Allahan & Côté, 1998; Yalnizyan, 1998; Armstrong, 1997; McDaniel, 1997) Virtually all of these programs are under threat, have been reduced, or transformed into targeted programs. Meanwhile new problems are emerging. The most obvious are HIV/AIDS and Alzheimer's.

One program under threat is the health-care system. Enormous changes have taken place in this system throughout the last one hundred years but the last decade has seen some of the most important for caregiving. New techniques, drugs and technologies have made it possible to do day surgery and provide many other interventions on an outpatient basis or with shorter patient stays. Moreover, many of the sophisticated treatments once available only within hospitals can now be done at home, thanks in part to new equipment. Combined with an emphasis on cost-cutting, these developments mean that many people are sent out of the hospital while still requiring complex and skilled care. The obvious consequence is more informal caregiving and unpaid caregivers providing much more complex care. The less obvious consequence is the entry into the home of strangers to assess the need for, and to provide, care. This can mean both less privacy and more conflict over what care is provided by whom. (Armstrong & Armstrong, 1996) And perhaps least obvious is the shifting of care costs onto the caregiver or recipient and their often shared concern about the quality of care provided by informal carers. It must be emphasized that this is not care being sent back home, where it was once done by mothers and daughters. Our grandmothers never cleaned catheters or checked intravenous tubes; they did not examine incisions or do much wound care.

Little research has been done on this new form of care but what is available indicates that the caregiving is done primarily by women. For elderly patients discharged early from hospital, access to formal in-home services were significant in boosting morale perhaps in part because they had confidence in the skills of the provider. (Chambers et al., 1990) In the case of patients recovering from cardiac surgery, 84 percent of the women caregivers were employed outside the home. Their jobs in "lower status positions" meant that leaves are difficult to obtain and caregiving, even for a short period, could threaten their jobs. (King & Koop, 1998)

The other, relatively recent development in health care is the move of people from institutions into the community. Deinstitutionalization began with psychiatric patients in the late 1960s (Simmons, 1990) and now applies to all those previously cared for in large facilities. Then, like now, the move has been made often without appropriate alternatives available and the community too often means a poorly-equipped home or the street. (Layton, 2000) Those at home are expected to provide care, and the expectations are higher for women. Moreover, such care often means giving up paid employment, and women are more likely to leave the labour force than men to provide care in part because they have the lower-paying jobs. (Statistics Canada, 2000) It may simply make sense, at least in the short term, for the lowest paid member to leave the labour force in order to provide necessary care and few jobs allow women to take paid leave to provide care.

This leads directly to another major change in women's labour force participation. Today, unlike a century ago, most women are in the labour force for most of their adult years. (Statistics Canada, 2000) They have jobs for many reasons, including the fact that jobs grew in traditional female work with the expansion of the welfare state. However, the single most important reason for taking paid work is the same for women and men: they need the income. (Statistics Canada, 2000) Although women have made significant progress within the labour force, they are still segregated into the lowest paid occupations. They are also over-represented in part-time and temporary work. Those who are self-employed seldom have people working for them and many hold multiple jobs. (Statistics Canada, 2000) Moreover, women's steady improvement since the 1950s seems to have halted or even reversed. "In 1999, 41 percent of employed women aged 15-64 had a non-standard employment arrangement, compared to 35 percent in 1989," and women's labour force participation rates have stayed virtually the same for the last decade. In that same year, 3 percent of women, compared to 1 percent of men in full-time jobs lost time at work because of family responsibilities. (Statistics Canada, 2000, 103) The increases in women's non-standard work may in part be explained by their increasing caregiving activities. Instead of losing time at work, they may have to take jobs that require less time or that can be done at home. Women's full-time work is less likely than men's to come with a private pension and non-standard work is even less likely to have any benefits at all. As a result, many of the women who account for the majority of the elderly have only public pensions. And for many, the lack of a pension is a direct result of their caregiving. (Townson, 1995)

At the same time, many of the employment protections have been removed in a deregulated market, leaving fewer and fewer households with even one secure, decently paid job to support the household.

Partly in response to these changes, more men and women are working longer hours often at two jobs. (Statistics Canada, 2000, 103) As a result, fewer and fewer families have the time or resources to provide much care just as care demands are increasing. This seems like a volatile mix.

There have also been changes in family patterns. There are fewer marriages and fewer children, born closer together in terms of age, within marriages. Openly common-law relationships have become much more common, as have openly gay and lesbian relationships. More marriages end in divorce and more blended families have children who still have other living parents outside the current marriage. (Ambert, 1998) More families have only one parent, most of them headed by women. Housing and job shortages, as well as inadequate incomes, are forcing more people to live with relatives and friends. And new patterns of immigration mean that households are much more culturally and racially diverse. (Wooley, 1998) What these developments mean for caregiving is difficult to determine but it is clear that the changes in relationships will influence where, when and how care can or will be provided. And it seems likely that there are fewer and fewer family members, and thus fewer people, to provide care.

4.3. The Changes That Matter For Care

What this summary indicates is that people have provided, and continue to provide, care for friends, relatives and strangers. For the most part, they do it willingly and with care. (Wolfson et al., 1993) Moreover, those who receive care now or in the past themselves provide care, and caregiving is often part of rewarding relationships. However, the demands on caregivers are expanding enormously with the increasing acuity and disability levels of those receiving informal care. Longevity is also contributing to the workload, although not as much as public discourse would suggest. Moreover, there are more people needing this complex care at the same time as the welfare state is reducing services provided in the formal system and increasing pressures on families in general and women in particular to fill the gaps. Yet more and more women have little choice but to work in the labour force, few of their labour force jobs allow them to provide care

The Commodity of Care   49

and, if they do give up full-time paid work in order to care, they are jeopardizing not only their future employment but also their money for old age as well. (Morris et al., 1999) More and more research is suggesting that this caregiving is often a burden under current conditions, placing strains not only on the health of the providers and recipients but also on their relationships and on both their current and future finances.

5. Framework for Assessing Legislation, Regulation, and Policy

This summary of 100 years of caregiving provides a basis for developing a framework for assessing government intervention. Legislation, regulation and social policy should seek to facilitate caregiving among adults, and do so in ways that allow both care providers and care recipients to retain their dignity and their relationships. This means asking the following questions:

1.   **Is caregiving and care receiving voluntary?** Caregiving can be voluntary only if there is access to alternatives and if there are the kinds of supports available that allow choices to be made. This, in turn, can mean the most effective and efficient care. The Hall Commission (Canada, 1964), which provided the basis for public health care, recommended that a full range of services, including homecare, long-term care and pharmacare, be publicly provided on the grounds that this would help ensure that services were delivered not only appropriately and in an accessible manner but also in the least expensive manner because choice would be based more on need than simply on what was available.

2.   **Can caregiving be equally shared among women and men?** Women told the National Forum on Health, a body established by Prime Minister Chretien to advise on the future of health care, that they did not want to be "conscripted" (National Forum on Health, 1997, 19) into unpaid caregiving. The research clearly shows that such caregiving is, and has been, primarily women's work. This is the case regardless of their age, income, labour force participation, cultural, physical or legal locations. While the values of the women who pro-

vide care play some role in this workload, there is significant evidence to demonstrate that legislation, regulations and policy constructs women as caregivers.

3. **Can caregiving be culturally sensitive without making inappropriate assumptions about cultural groups and without contravening other equity principles?** Equity, if defined as exactly the same services provided to everyone, can mean services that do not respond to many people's specific needs. Experience with both the *Canada Health Act* and the *Canadian Human Rights Act* has shown that it is possible to establish principles that allow for considerable variety in how these principles are met. There is considerable diversity in the needs, in the resources and desires of caregivers and recipients that should be, when appropriate, accommodated in legislation.

4. **Can the assumptions made about personal relationships related to caregiving be justified?** Legislation, regulations and policy often assume the heterosexual nuclear family. They also often assume that especially the women in such families have the skills, resources, time and desire to provide care. Yet many people do not live in such relationships, and those that do may not see their families as the best place to find or give care. Equally important, caregiving often involves many people with no blood or marital ties who nevertheless need supports in order to provide care

5. **Is there recognition of the different interests that need to be balanced in caregiving?** In searching for ways to facilitate caregiving, it is necessary to recognize that there are tensions and differences that can never be resolved, but rather need to be balanced and understood in their particular contexts. Perhaps the most critical of these is the tension between care providers and care recipient. Each has different, and often contradictory, needs. Paid and unpaid providers also frequently have conflicting practices and agendas. So too do governments and institutions focused on costs savings when they encounter caregivers seeking supports. There are also tensions between the desire for privacy and the need for caregivers to share information; be-

tween the transfer of care to the private home and the regular entry into that home of care providers. All these, and more, tensions exist within the larger one between individual and collective responsibility for care.

6. **Is need defined in ways that exclude some groups while privileging or stigmatizing others?** Programs and supports defined as welfare rather than as universal rights can serve to create inequalities. As the discussions and research that led to many social programs in Canada make clear, we are all at risk of illness and disability, and thus in need of care. Illness is usually not the fault of the individual and frail old age is seldom attributable to individual actions. Canadians have agreed that we have a collective responsibility for care and that care is a right, not a privilege. It is important for legislation, regulations and policy to reflect this right.

7. **What are the long-term consequences?** Although some services and supports and obligations may seem to make sense today, they may have negative consequences in the future. So, for example, a woman who provides care for her partner may benefit immediately from a caregiver allowance but this allowance may mean she drops out of the labour force and finds herself in poverty when she is old. Moreover, the care she provides today may cut her off from friends who will provide her with support tomorrow. In thinking about consequences, we need to think beyond the provider and recipients to their network of relationships and to the larger society.

8. **Are the objectives reinforced or undermined by other legislation, regulations or policy?** Strategies in one sector may enable caregiving while those in another may mean caregiving is a burden. For example flexible hours in paid work may allow women to be caregivers at home or in their community but they may also serve to reinforce women's responsibility for this caregiving, limiting their capacity to do their paid work or threatening their health. Or respite services available for caregivers may be out of reach because there is no accessible public transit to the care. Or housing policies may mean

that people who need some care cannot afford to live in their own homes or independently.

9. **Are the contributions of care recipients recognized and the skills required for giving care acknowledged?** While the research shows that care recipients are often the most vulnerable and in need of complex services, it also shows that many care recipients are themselves contributors in forms of caregiving. It is important to recognize their participation and facilitate it. It is just as important to recognize that care is skilled work, especially as more and more complex care needs are sent home.

10. **Are current patterns themselves constructs of policy or does policy reflect actual preferences and practices?** It is important to ask if policies have created patterns that then get replicated in ways that exclude alternatives. For example, current immigrant laws on family unification mean that those families that want to live with relatives are the most likely to apply and, in any case, the regulations require these families to continue supporting the relatives brought into Canada under these provisions. It cannot be assumed that families who immigrate under such conditions reflect all families from these cultures, however, or that these families have the resources necessary to provide such care.

Concluding Remarks

The research on unpaid caregiving suggests "the need to refocus attention away from the creation of partnerships and protecting against unnecessary substitution towards broader concerns with supporting the partnerships that already exists." (Penning, 2000, 76) The risk is not that families will not provide care but rather that they will not be able to provide care without risking their health and their relationships if formal services fail to support them. Indeed, "more generous social programs reinforce both family and social responsibility." (Baker, 1996, 3) Under conditions of declining public support, broader definitions of family may simply mean more people are conscripted into care rather than better caregiving or better relationships. Unless there are formal supports for unpaid caregiving, both the caregivers and their relationships are increasingly likely to fall apart. And such supports need to recognize the diversity in needs and the diversity in networks, networks that extend beyond kin to create the most satisfying care. (Stewart, 2000)

Bibliography

Allahan, A.L. & J.E. Côté (1998). *Richer and Poorer, the Structure of Inequality in Canada*, Toronto, Lorimer.

Ambert, A.-M. (1998). *Divorce: Facts, Figures and Consequences*, Ottawa, The Vanier Institute of the Family.

Armstrong, Pat (1997). "The Welfare State as History," in R.B. Blake, P. Bryden and J.F. Strain (eds.), *The Welfare State in Canada. Past, Present and Future*, Concord, Ontario, Irwin Publishers.

Armstrong, Pat & Hugh Armstrong (1999). *Women, Privatization and Health Care Reform: The Ontario Case*, Toronto, National Network on Environments and Women's Health.

Armstrong, Pat & Hugh Armstrong (1998). *Universal Health Care: What the U.S. Can Learn from the Canadian Experience*, New York, New Press.

Armstrong, Pat & Hugh Armstrong (1996). *Wasting Away: The Undermining of Canadian Health Care*, Toronto, Oxford University Press.

Armstrong, Pat & Hugh Armstrong (1994). *The Double Ghetto. Canadian Women and Their Segregated Work*, 3rd ed., Toronto, Oxford University Press.

Aronson, Jane (1998). "Women's Perspectives on Informal Care of the Elderly: Public Ideology and Personal Experience of Giving and Receiving Care." in David Coburn, C. D'Arcy and George Torrance (eds.), *Health and Canadian Society: Sociological Perspectives*, Toronto, University of Toronto Press.

Aronson, Jane (1990). "Old Women's Experiences of Needing Care: Choice or Compulsion?" *Canadian Journal on Aging/La Revue Canadienne du Vieillissement*, 9:3.

Aronson, Jane & Sheila Neysmith (1997). "The Retreat of the State and Long-Term Provision: Implementations for Frail Elderly People, Unpaid Family Carers and Paid Home-Care Workers," *Studies in Political Economy*, 53.

Bacovsky, R. (1997). *Federal, Provincial and Territorial Government Sponsored Drug Plans and Drug Databases: Background Information Prepared for the Conference on National Approaches to Pharmacare.*

Bailey, M. (2000). "Foreword," *Canadian Journal of Family Law*, 17:1.

Baker, M. (1996). *Reinforcing Obligations and Responsibilities between Generations: Policy Options from Cross-National Comparisons*, Ottawa, The Vanier Institute of the Family.

Banting, Keith (1982). *The Welfare State and Canadian Federalism*, Kingston, Brown & Martin.

Bernier, J. & M. Dallaire (2000). *What Price Have Women Paid for Health Care Reform? The Situation in Québec*, Montréal, Le Centre d'excellence pour la santé des femmes-Consortium, Université de Montréal.

Blackie, N.K. et al. (1985). *Innovations in Housing and Living Arrangements for Seniors*, Burnaby, B.C., Gerontology Research Centre, Simon Fraser University.

Blakley, B.M. & J. Jaffe (1999). *Coping as a Rural Caregiver: The Impact of Health Care Reforms on Rural Women Informal Caregivers*. http://www.pwhce.ca/swan.htm

Bracci, C. (2000). "Ties That Bind: Ontario's *Filial Responsibility Act*." *Canadian Journal of Family Law*, 17:2.

Bradbury, B. (1993). *Working Families: Age, Gender, and Daily Survival in Industrializing Montreal*, Toronto, McClelland & Stewart.

Brotman, S. (1998). "The Incidence of Poverty Among Seniors in Canada: Exploring the Impact of Gender, Ethnicity and Race," *Canadian Journal on Aging/ La Revue Canadienne du Vieillissement*, 17:2.

Buchignani, N. & C. Armstrong-Esther (1999). "Informal Care and Older Native Canadians," *Ageing and Society*, 19:1, 3-32.

Campbell, L.D. & A. Martin-Matthews (2000). "Caring Sons: Exploring Men's Involvement in Filial Care," *Canadian Journal on Aging/La Revue Canadienne du Vieillissement*, 1.

Canada (2000). *Agreement between the Treasury Board and the Professional Institute of the Public Service of Canada*, Treasury Board of Canada. http://www.tbs.sct.gc.ca/Pubs_pol/hrpubs/coll_agre/sh_e.html

Canada (1996). *Employment Insurance Act, S.C. 1996, c.23.*

Canada, (1964). *Report of the Royal Commission on Health Services*, Ottawa, Queen's Printer.

CMHC (1983). *Housing the Elderly*, Ottawa, Canada Mortgage and Housing Corporation.

CHCA (1998). Canadian Home Care Association (in collaboration with L'Association des CLSC et des CHSLD du Quebec), *Portrait of Canada: An Overview of Public Home Care Programs*, Ottawa, Health Canada.

Chambers, L. et al. (1990). "Impact of Home Care on Recently Discharged Elderly Hospital Patients in an Ontario Community," *Canadian Journal on Aging/La Revue Canadienne du Vieillissement*, 9:4.

Chappell, N. & A. Blandford (1991). "Informal and Formal Care: Exploring the Complementarity," *Ageing and Society*, 11 (Part 3).

Chappell, N. & M.J. Prince (1997). "Reasons Why Canadian Seniors Volunteer," *Canadian Journal on Aging/La Revue Canadienne du Vieillissement*, 16:2.

Chappell, N., L.A. Strain & A.A. Blandford (1986). *Aging and Health Care : A Social Perspective*, Toronto, Holt, Rinehart and Winston of Canada.

Che-Alford, J. & B. Hamm (1999). "Under One Roof: Three Generations Living Together," *Canadian Social Trends*, Summer.

J. Chen & R. Wilkins (1998). "Seniors' Needs for Health-Related Personal Assistance," *Health Reports*, 10:11.

Chubachi, N. (1999). *Geographies of Nisei Japanese Canadians and Their Attitudes Towards Elderly Long-Term Care*, M.A. thesis, Queen's University, Ontario.

Cloutier-Fisher, D. & A.E. Joseph (2000). "Long-Term Care Restructuring in Rural Ontario: Retrieving Community Service User and Provider Narratives," *Social Science and Medicine*, 50, 7-8.

Cochrane, J.J. , P.N. Goering & J.M. Rogers (1997). "The Mental Health of Informal Caregivers in Ontario: An Epidemiological Survey," *American Journal of Public Health*, 87:12.

Cohen, M.G. (1988). *Women's Work, Markets, and Economic Development in Nineteenth-Century Ontario*, Toronto, University of Toronto Press.

Colantonio, A., C. Cohen & S. Corlett (1998). "Support Needs of Elderly Caregivers of Persons with Dementia," *Canadian Journal on Aging/La Revue Canadienne du Vieillissement*, 17:3.

Connidis, I.A. (1983). "Living Arrangement Choices of Older Residents,"*Canadian Journal of Sociology/Cahiers canadiens de sociologie*, 8.

Cott, C.A. & M.A.M. Gignac (1999). "Independence and Dependence for Older Adults with Osteoarthritis or Osteoporosis." *Canadian Journal on Aging/ La Revue Canadienne du Vieillissement*, 18:1.

Cranswick, K. (1999). "Help Close at Hand: Relocating to Give or Receive Care," *Canadian Social Trends*.

Crompton, S. & A. Kemeny (1999). "In Sickness and in Health: The Well-Being of Married Seniors," *Canadian Social Trends*.

Dalley, G. (1988). *Ideologies of Caring : Rethinking Community and Collectivism*, Basingstoke, Macmillan Education.

Davies, L. et al. (2001). *Social Policy, Gender Inequality and Poverty*, Ottawa, Status of Women Canada.

Davies, M.J. (forthcoming). *Into the House of the Old: A History of Residential Care in B.C.*, unpublished manuscript.

Denton, Margaret (1997). "The Linkages between Informal and Formal Care of the Elderly," *Canadian Journal on Aging/La Revue Canadienne du Vieillissement*, 16:1.

Dhawan, S. (1998). *Caregiving Stress and Acculturation in East Indian Immigrants: Caring for Their Elders*, Ph.D thesis, Queen's University, Ontario.

Dillon, L. (forthcoming). "Elderly Women in Late Victorian Canada," in B. Hesketh and C. Hackett, eds., *Canada: Confederation to Present* (CD-Rom), University of Alberta.

Dillon, L. (1998). "Parent-Child Co-Residence among the Elderly in 1871 Canada and 1880 United States: A Comparative Study," in E.-A. Montigny and A.L. Chambers, eds., *Family Matters: Papers in Post-Confederation Canadian Family History*, Toronto, Canadian Scholars' Press.

Dorazio-Migliore, M. (1999). *Eldercare in Context: Narrative, Gender, and Ethnicity*, Ph.D. thesis, University of British Columbia.

Doyle, V.M. (1989). *Homesharing Matchup Agencies for Seniors : A Literature Review*, Burnaby, B.C., Gerontology Research Centre, Simon Fraser University.

Echenberg, H. (1998). *Income Security and Support for Persons with Disabilities: Future Directions*, Ottawa, Canadian Labour Congress.

Eichler, M. (2000). "Contemporary and Historical Diversity in Families: Comment on Turcotte's and Smart's Papers," *Canadian Journal of Family Law*, 17:2.

Esteves, E. (2000). "The New Wageless Worker: Volunteering and Market-Guided Health Care Reform," in D.L. Gustafson, ed., *Care and Consequences. The Impact of Health Care Reform*, Halifax, Fernwood Publishing.

Finch, J. & D. Groves (1983). *A Labour of Love : Women, Work, and Caring*, London, Routledge & K. Paul.

Frederick, J.A. & J.E. Fast (1999). "Eldercare in Canada: Who Does How Much?" *Canadian Social Trends*.

Fuller, Colleen (1999). *Reformed or Rerouted? Women and Change in the Health Care System*, Vancouver, British Columbia Centre of Excellence for Women's Health.

Gignac, M.A.M., E.K. Kelloway & B.H. Gottlieb (1996). "Impact of Caregiving on Employment: A Mediational Model of Work-Family Conflict," *Canadian Journal on Aging/La Revue Canadienne du Vieillissement*, 15:4.

Guest, Dennis (1980). *The Emergence of Social Security in Canada*, Vancouver, University of British Columbia Press.

Gurevich, M. (1999). *Privatization in Health Reform from Women's Perspectives: Research, Policy and Responses*, Halifax, Maritime Centre of Excellence for Women's Health.

Gutman, G.M. (1995). *Literature Review: Characteristics, Service Needs and Service Preferences of Younger Adults with Severe Physical Disabilities*, Burnaby, Gerontology Research Centre, Simon Fraser University.

Gutman, G.M. (1989). *Survey of Canadian Homesharing Agencies Serving the Elderly*. Burnaby, Gerontology Research Centre, Simon Fraser University.

Gutman, G.M. & N.K. Blackie (1988). *Housing the Very Old*, Burnaby, Gerontology Research Centre, Simon Fraser University.

Jenson, Jane & S. Jacobzone (2000). *Care Allowances for the Frail Elderly and Their Impact on Women Care-Givers*, Paris, Organization for Economic Co-operation and Development. Directorate for Education Employment Labour and Social Affairs.

Keating, N.C., J. Fast, J. Frederick (1999). *Eldercare in Canada: Context, Content and Consequences*, Ottawa, Statistics Canada.

Keefe, J.M. & P. Fancey (1997). "Financial Compensation or Home Help Services: Examining Differences among Program Recipients," *Canadian Journal on Aging/La Revue Canadienne du Vieillissement*, 16:2.

King, K.M. & P.M. Koop (1999). "The Influence of the Cardiac Surgery Patient's Sex and Age on Care-Giving Received,"*Social Science and Medicine*, 48:12.

Kobayashi, K.M. (2000). *The Nature of Support from Adult Sansei (Third Generation) Children to Older Nisei (Second Generation) Parents in Japanese Canadian Families*, Hamilton, McMaster University, SEDAP Research Paper No. 18.

Lavoie, J.-P. (1995). "Support Groups for Informal Caregivers Don't Work! Refocus the Groups or the Evaluations?" *Canadian Journal on Aging/La Revue Canadienne du Vieillissement*, 14:3.

Layton, Jack (2000). *Homelessness: The Making and Unmaking of a Crisis*, Toronto, Penguin.

Lindsay, C. (1999). "Seniors: A Diverse Group Aging Well," *Canadian Social Trends*.

MacBride-King, J.L. (1999). *Caring About Caregiving: The Eldercare Responsibilites of Canadian Workers and the Impact on Employers*, Ottawa, The Conference Board of Canada.

Marsh, Leonard (1975). *Report on Social Security for Canada*, with a new introduction by the author and a preface by Michael Bliss, Toronto, University of Toronto Press.

McCann, K. & E. Wadsworth (1992). "The Role of Informal Carers in Supporting Gay Men Who Have HIV Related Illness," *AIDS Care*, 4:1.

McDaniel, S. & R. Lewis (1998). "Did They or Didn't They? Intergeneration Supports in Families Past: A Case Study of Brigus, Newfoundland, 1920-1945," in E.-A. Montigny and A.L. Chambers, eds., *Family Matters: Papers in Post-Confederation Canadian Family History*, Toronto, Canadian Scholars' Press.

McDaniel, S.A. (1997). "Serial Employment and Skinny Government: Reforming Caring and Sharing Among Generations," *Canadian Journal on Aging/La Revue Canadienne du Vieillissement*, 16:3.

McGilly, F. (1991). *An Introduction to Canada's Public Social Services: Understanding Income and Health Programs*, Toronto, McClelland & Stewart.

Meshefedjian, G. et al. (1998). "Factors Associated with Symptoms of Depression among Informal Caregivers of Demented Elders in the Community," *Gerontologist*, 38 (2).

Montigny, E.A. (2000). "Families, Institutions, and the State in Late-Nineteenth-Century Ontario," in E.-A. Montigny and A.L. Chambers, eds., *Ontario since Confederation: A Reader*, Toronto, University of Toronto Press.

Montigny, E.A. (1997). *Foisted Upon the Government? State Responsibilities, Family Obligations, and the Care of the Dependent Aged in Late Nineteenth-Century Ontario*, Montreal, McGill-Queen's University Press.

Montigny , E.-A. & A.L. Chambers (eds.) (1998). *Family Matters: Papers in Post-Confederation Canadian Family History*, Toronto, Canadian Scholars' Press.

Moore, H. (1997). *Caregiving in Parkinson's: A Qualitative Study of the Perceived Impacts on and Needs of Parkinson's Caregivers*, M.Sc. thesis, Queen's University, Ontario.

Morris, M. et al. (1999). *The Changing Nature of Home Care and Its Impact on Women's Vulnerability to Poverty*, Ottawa, Status of Women Canada.

Morrongiello, B. & B. Gottlieb (2000). "Self-Care among Adults," *Canadian Journal on Aging/La Revue Canadienne du Vieillissement*, 19:1.

Myles, John (2000). "The Maturation of Canada's Retirement Income System: Income Levels, Income Inequality and Low Income among Older Persons," *Canadian Journal on Aging/La Revue Canadienne du Vieillissement*, 19:3.

National Forum on Health (1997). *Canada Health Action: Building on the Legacy. Synthesis Report and Issues Papers*, Ottawa, Public Works and Government Services.

Neysmith, Sheila (2000). *Restructuring Caring Labour: Discourse, State Practice, and Everyday Life*, Toronto, Oxford University Press.

Ontario Human Rights Commission (2000). *Discrimination and Age*, Toronto, Ontario Human Rights Commission.

Ontario (1991). Ministry of Community and Social Services, *Redirection of Long-Term Care and Support Service in Ontario*, Toronto, Queen's Printer for Ontario.

O'Rourke, N. et al. (1996). "Relative Contribution of Subjective Factors to Expressed Burden among Spousal Caregivers of Suspected Dementia Patients," *Canadian Journal on Aging/La Revue Canadienne du Vieillissement*, 15:4.

Parr, J. (1995). *A Diversity of Women: Ontario, 1945-1980*, Toronto, University of Toronto Press.

Parr, J. (1990). *The Gender of Breadwinners: Women, Men, and Change in Two Industrial Towns, 1880-1950*, Toronto, University of Toronto Press.

Penning, M.J. (2000), "Self-, Informal and Formal Care: Partnerships in Community-Based and Residential Long-Term Settings," *Canadian Journal on Aging/La Revue Canadienne du Vieillissement*, 19 (Supplement 1).

Porter, John (1965). *The Vertical Mosaic*, Toronto, University of Toronto Press.

Robb, R. et al. (1999). "Valuation of Unpaid Help by Seniors in Canada: An Empirical Analysis," *Canadian Journal on Aging/La Revue Canadienne du Vieillissement*, 18:4.

Rosenberg, M.W. & E.G. Moore (1997). "The Health of Canada's Elderly Population: Current Status and Future Implications," *Canadian Medical Association Journal*, 157.

Rosenthal, C.J. & A. Martin-Matthews (1999). *Families as Care-Providers Versus Care-Managers? Gender and Type of Care in a Sample of Employed Canadians*, Hamilton, McMaster University, Sedap Research Paper No. 4.

Rosenthal, C.J.& L.O. Stone (1999). *How Much Help Is Exchanged in Families? Towards an Understanding of Discrepant Research Findings*, Hamilton, McMaster University, SEDAP Research Paper No. 2.

Salvatori, P. et al. (1998). "Aging with an Intellectual Disability: A Review of Canadian Literature," *Canadian Journal on Aging/La Revue Canadienne du Vieillissement*, 17:3.

Sauvé, R. (1999). *The Current State of Canadian Family Finances 1999 Report*, Ottawa, The Vanier Institute of the Family.

Simmons, H.G. (1990). *Unbalanced : Mental Health Policy in Ontario, 1930-1989*, Toronto, Wall & Thompson.

Smart, C. (2000). "Stories of Family Life: Cohabitation, Marriage and Social Change," *Canadian Journal of Family Law*, 17:1.

Snell, J.G. (1996). *The Citizen's Wage: The State and the Elderly in Canada, 1900-1951*, Toronto, University of Toronto Press.

Snell, J.G. (1990). "Filial Responsibility Laws in Canada: An Historical Study," *Canadian Journal on Aging/La Revue Canadienne du Vieillissement*, 9:3.

Spencer, C., M. Ashfield & A. Vanderbijl (1996). *Abuse and Neglect of Older Adults in Community Settings: An Annotated Bibliography*, Burnaby, Gerontology Research Centre, Simon Fraser University.

Statistics Canada (2000). *Women in Canada 2000*, Ottawa, Ministry of Industry.

Statistics Canada (1998). *Caring Canadians, Involved Canadians: Highlights from the 1997 National Survey of Giving, Volunteering and Participating*, Ottawa, Statistics Canada.

Statistics Canada (1997). "Who Cares? Caregiving in the 1990's," The Daily.

Stewart, M. (2000). *Chronic Conditions and Caregiving in Canada : Social Support Strategies*, Toronto, University of Toronto Press.

Struthers, James (1994). *The Limits of Affluence: Welfare in Ontario, 1920-1970*, Toronto, University of Toronto Press.

Taylor, D. (forthcoming). "Making Care Visible: Exploring the Healthwork of People Living with HIVAIDS in Ontario."

Taylor, Malcolm (1978). *Health Insurance and Canadian Public Policy*, Kingston, McGill-Queen's University Press.

The Roeher Institute (2001). *Personal Relationships of Support between Adults: The Case of Disability*, Toronto, The Roeher Institute.

Vanier Institute (n.d.). *The Family. From the Kitchen Table to the Boardroom Table. A Digest*, Ottawa, The Vanier Institute of the Family.

Townson, Monica, *Women's Financial Futures: Mid-Life Prospects for a Secure Retirement*, Ottawa, Canadian Advisory Council on the Status of Women.

Trottier, H. et al. (2000). "Living at Home or in an Institution: What Makes the Difference for Seniors?" *Health Reports.* 11:4.

Ward-Griffin, C. (1998). *Negotiating the Boundaries of Eldercare: The Relationship between Nurses and Family Caregivers*, Ph.D. thesis, University of Toronto.

Ward-Griffin, C. & P. McKeever (2000). "Relationships between Nurses and Family Caregivers: Partners in Care?" *Advances in Nursing Science*, 22:3.

Wilkins, K. & M.P. Beaudet (2000). "Changes in Social Support in Relation to Seniors' Use of Home Care," *Health Reports*, 11:4, 39.

Wilson, K. & J. Howard (2000). *Missing Links: The Effects of Health Care Privatization on Women in Manitoba and Saskatchewan*, Winnipeg, Prairie Women's Health Centre of Excellence.

Wolfson, C. (1993). "Adult Children's Perceptions of Their Responsibility to Provide Care for Dependent Elderly Parents," *Gerontologist*, 33:3.

Wooley, Frances (1998). *Work and Household Transactions: An Economist's View*, Ottawa, Canadian Policy Research Networks.

Yalnizyan, Armine (1998). *The Growing Gap: A Report on Growing Inequality Between the Rich and the Poor in Canada*, Toronto, Centre for Social Justice.

Note

[1]   An earlier version of this chapter was prepared for the Law Commission of Canada under the title *One Hundred Years of Caregiving* The views expressed are those of the authors and do not necessarily reflect the views of the Commission. The accuracy of the information contained in the paper is the sole responsibility of the authors.

Chapter 2
Responding to State Retrenchment:
An Historical Perspective on Non-Profit Home
Health and Social Care in Ontario
Tamara J. Daly[1]

1. Introduction

Policy makers have embraced the idea that the non-profit sector can play an expanded role in building and maintaining strong communities. Hall and Banting (2000) suggest that the voluntary sector "…appears to be emerging as a chosen instrument of collective action in the new century." In Ontario, the Advisory Board on the Voluntary Sector (1997) stated that "[n]otwithstanding government rationalization at all levels, governments have a responsibility to provide a policy, legislative and regulatory environment that facilitates and supports voluntary organizations and voluntary action." Yet, government retrenchment since the early 1990s has led to a reduction in the availability of many government-funded community and social services. (Hall & Banting, 2000) Calling for an expanded role for voluntary non-profit organizations is difficult in a situation dominated by government rationalization and retrenchment. It ignores the historical reality that "…government has always been a pervasive influence in the activities of the voluntary sector (even prior to the mid 1980s), although the extent of that influence has not been emphasized." (Hall & Reed, 1998) More and more, organizations are involved in providing services once delivered directly by the state while their ability to deliver complementary services has declined. Speaking against the downloading that Canadian governments have engaged in, Neil Brooks argues:

> [v]oluntary organizations should complement government activity, not substitute for it. Calling on the voluntary sector

to replace government services threatens the characteristics that provide its strengths and that constitute its unique attributes as a form of social organization, such as flexibility, responsiveness to local and minority interests, the capacity to innovate and initiate new ideas, and the ability to oversee and monitor the exercise of power by the state and other dominating institutions in society. (Brooks, 1999, 166)

Over the past two decades, increasing attention has been paid to the role of the voluntary non-profit sector in many countries, including Canada, the United States and the United Kingdom. A 1997 OECD report declares that governments will increasingly cease to engage in activities that may be "...delegated to regional, municipal, cooperative, mutualist or private organizations...letting citizens themselves—and no longer cold and distant bureaucracies—devise 'neighbourhood' solutions for everything pertaining to education, the fight against poverty, exclusion, drug trades, taking care of the young, dynamizing a local environment, etc." (OECD, 1997) In Canada, policy documents, speeches and reports produced since the 1970s are replete with references to the contribution that voluntary organizations can make to reinvigorate the role of government. These documents often ignore the critical role government has historically played in the development and growth of the non-profit sector, and the damage inflicted on the latter by the withdrawal of state support.

In the past, Ontario has at different times and in different ways encouraged the proliferation of non-profit organizations in the home-health-and-social-care sector. During the first half of the twentieth century, non-profit organizations were quite autonomous from the state; they provided home health and social care thanks to a mixture of private philanthropy and inconsistent public grants. By the late 1950s and early 1960s, they had begun to play an important role in the provision of state-funded health services, relying on a combination of formal state grants and limited charitable donations. As government committees called for restraint in provincial public spending in the 1970s, outsourcing services to non-profit and other private organizations became an entrenched practice. With the recent rise of the state as "contractor, regulator and partner" (Stein, 2001), the traditional boundaries dividing the state, the market and non-profit organizations have been re-drawn. Non-profit organizations now provide home-care services as sub-contractors of the state within a market environment. Since 1995, the Ministry of Health and Long Term Care (MOHLTC) has established two types of contract models for home health and social care:

- the competitive tendering of home-care-service contracts for professional and paraprofessional home-care services—managed competition; and
- a "quasi" fee-for-service contract model for community-support services.

A number of analysts have noted that reform of the home-care system has had an impact on non-profit organizations (Jenson & Phillips, 2000; Baranek et al, 1999); others have looked at the evolving relationship between the state and the non-profit sector in the U.S. (Salamon, 1995) and Canada. (Brooks, 1999; Hall & Reed, 1998; Browne, 1996; Rekart, 1993) Building on their insights, I argue that the state has changed the foundations upon which many non-profits were built. Its imposition of a "culture of efficiency and accountability" (Stein, 2001) has changed its relationship with them. They no longer feel they are partners, but rather contractors, and sometimes providers of last resort. To be viable they must also be able to compete for home-care contracts with private businesses. This has jeopardized their stability.

Rice and Prince (2000) argue that the shift to a mixed welfare state involves two forms of state retrenchment. *Systemic retrenchment* shifts overall institutional and fiscal practices, with implications for the overall political environment (e.g., interest group behaviour, public opinion, inter-governmental relations and government finances).[2] (Rice & Prince, 2000; Pierson, 1994) *Programmatic retrenchment* involves cutting the amount of expenditures, inserting more or different rules and regulations into the design of programs, and making programs a residual, last resort—after private markets and families fail. (Rice & Prince, 2000; Pierson, 1994) While both forms of retrenchment are a part of recent home-care reform, I shall focus mainly on the impact of programmatic retrenchment on non-profit organizations, as evidenced in the shifting nature of home-care services and public funding.[3]

Some Definitions

Long-term care is a continuum along which many different types of clients, providers, and funding mechanisms come together in a variety of settings: chronic-care hospitals, nursing homes, supportive housing, private residences. I shall focus specifically on home care, defined as: "an array of services which enable clients, incapacitated in whole or in part, to live at home, often with the effect of preventing, delaying, or substituting for long-term care or acute care alternatives." (Health Canada, 1990) In Ontario, the *Long Term Care Act, 1994* (Bill 173) defined four categories of publicly funded home-care services:

- *Professional services* include nursing, rehabilitation therapies, nutrition, and social work. They are provided by licensed professionals.
- *Personal support services* include bathing, dressing, lifting etc. In Ontario, personal support workers are licensed through a community college program (or the equivalent).
- *Homemaking* includes services such as cleaning, vacuuming, and laundry. Homemakers are not licensed, but are usually bonded. They work across the continuum, in for-profit and non-profit professional and personal support organizations, or with community-based non-profit organizations as staff or on a contract basis.
- Finally, *community support services* include meals-on-wheels, friendly visiting, home help, home maintenance and repair, security checks, and transportation (Figure 1). The staff, contract workers and volunteers of community-support non-profit organizations and municipalities provide these services.

Under the *Canada Health Act, 1984*, insured services, such as those provided by hospitals and physicians, are free and universally accessible on the basis of medical necessity. Long-term care has elements of both social care and health care. In Ontario, home-care services partly

Figure 1

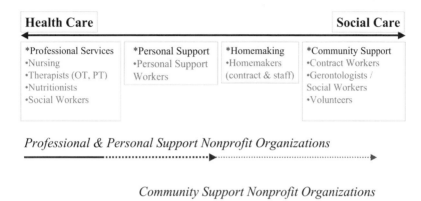

developed within the logic of universally accessible health care; however, eligibility for care may also be based on factors such as risk of institutionalization, isolation, and frailty, that may not be considered issues of medical necessity. Clients are typically charged user fees for many such services (although some are free); payment is based on means testing.

The home-health-and-social-care sector comprises two main *types* of non-profit organization (although, in reality, the distinctions between the different types of organization are not always as clearly delineated):

- *professional and paraprofessional organizations* that have contracts with the Community Care Access Centres (CCACs) to provide services such as nursing, homemaking, physiotherapy, occupational therapy, speech therapy, nutrition (the MOHLTC refers collectively to the non-profit and for-profit organizations providing these services through contract with CCACs as *vendor agencies*);
- *community support organizations* organizations that receive provincial-government funding directly to provide services such as meals-on-wheels, friendly visiting, home help, home maintenance

and repair, security checks, and transportation (the MOHLTC refers to these organizations as *transfer of payments agencies*).

2. A Brief History of Non-Profit Organizations in Ontario Home Care

Providers of Last Resort (Before 1945)

In early Canada, there were three major access points for health and social care:

- the informal system of care provided by family, friends and neighbours;
- voluntary non-profit organizations for those who needed more help than could be provided by informal care networks;
- and finally the private market for those who could afford to pay for services. (Rice and Prince, 2000)

Many voluntary non-profit organizations were rooted in religious or ethnic communities. These organizations operated, in effect, as providers of last resort. Even though there was a greater separation between the state and voluntary organizations than in the present period, voluntary organizations still relied on government funding to address critical needs. Guest argues that this fragmented approach to social services fostered a "crisis approach" to the provision of social services. (Guest, 1986)

In the 1791 legislation creating Upper Canada (which later became Ontario) and Lower Canada (which later became Quebec), English common law continued to apply in Upper Canada; however, the Elizabethan Poor Law of 1601 was not retained (Mishra, Laws & Harding, 1988; Moscovitch & Drover, 1987).[4] This critical policy decision defined the nature of the voluntary non-profit sector to this day. The omission of the Poor Law provisions from the legislation creating Upper Canada was important for three reasons:

1. The omission left open the possibility of locating responsibility for at least some aspects of health and social welfare under the auspices of the state.

2. It also enabled other non-religiously affiliated organizations to have equal standing with religious organizations in the provision of social welfare services.
3. It maintained an existing role for the provision of care for the needy within the private sphere and outside of the public, state sphere.

Ontario's 1874 Charity Aid Act institutionalized the state's role in providing grants to private charities, conditional upon the imposition of certain regulations.

The British North America Act of 1867, which created Canada, divided powers between the federal government and the provinces, conferring on provincial legislatures exclusive power for the "Establishment, Maintenance and Management of Hospitals, Asylums, Charities, and Eleemosynary Institutions in the Province, other than Marine Hospitals." The specification of provincial power over hospitals had an important channeling effect on future federal government involvement in health care. In the mid-1900s, the federal government was ruled *ultra vires* in some of its attempts to extend its role in health care, as the latter was deemed to fall squarely within provincial jurisdiction under the constitution.

During the nineteenth century, the expansion of industrialization and urbanization began to expose underlying social problems in Ontario. Modernizing forces including social mobility, urbanization, individualism and market dependence destroyed pre-industrial modes of social reproduction, for example the role played by both the church and the family. These modernizing forces resulted in the absorption of the tasks of welfare by the modern nation state. (Flora & Alber, 1981) However, there was, in fact, a noticeable lag between the development of large-scale state involvement in social policy and the destruction of pre-industrial modes of social reproduction, such that it is difficult to explain the creation of the welfare state solely in terms of the failure of market forces to assume responsibility for welfare. (Esping-Andersen, 1990) Esping-Andersen points out that this theory of the expansion of state involvement in welfare does not adequately account for why government social policy emerged fifty, and sometimes one hundred, years after traditional community was dismantled. While large-scale state-sponsored social policies would not emerge until the middle of the century, it was during this early period that both lay and religious organizations' lobbying of government led to the first movement to expand the funding and delivery of social-welfare services by the state. This initial expansion stands in contrast to the argument that the state was absent from social policy in early nineteenth-century Canada when modernizing forces were pervasive. It was the involvement of both the municipal and provincial governments in the funding and delivery of these social-welfare services that formally institutionalized a role for both levels of governments in social services. For instance, the state expanded its reach into the provision of provincial and municipal institutional facilities such as asylums, institutions for the mentally ill, schools for the deaf and blind, as well as homes for the aged. (Mishra et al., 1988) Later, the passage of legislation to protect children's welfare (the *Children's Protection Act* of 1893) led to the creation of the Children's Aid Society, a partnership between a non-profit voluntary organization and the state.

Despite the involvement of the state in the funding and delivery of social services, most of the initiative during this period came from voluntary and philanthropic endeavours. The state played a minimal role, with local and/or provincial government authorities operating one set of institutions, while another was run by voluntary non-profit agencies (either religious or secular) usually with funding from the state. (Bellamy, 1983) Despite the involvement of the provincial and local levels of government in funding voluntary agencies to deliver services, it was not until the social-welfare crisis brought about by the Great Depression of the 1930s that the provincial and federal governments began to spend much more on support for the poor and social welfare more generally. The expansion of the state's role in funding the service-delivery capacity of voluntary non-profit health organizations for social welfare grew steadily from the 1930s until 1945.

Partners in State Expansion (1945 – mid-1970s)

The Canadian welfare state developed out of the compromise that followed World War II. Two dominant ideas combined to mould the general policy direction:

- the *moral* ideal of a Beveridge-style, universal, general-revenue-financed system espousing equality of status. (Taylor, 1987)
- the *economic* model of Keynesian demand-side economics, which provided the impetus for the expansion of the federal state into funding and the delivery of income security, health, social welfare, education and housing programs. (Jenson, 1989)

The size of expenditures on social welfare programs grew enormously during this period, prompting Lang to refer to this period as characterized by the emergence of a "service state" in Ontario. (Lang, 1974) Ontario's expenditures on health, education and welfare escalated rapidly, ballooning from just less than four percent (3.8) of Gross Provincial Product in 1946 to just over thirteen percent (13.1) by 1971. (Lang, 1974)

Throughout this period, the federal government offered the provinces funding to run programs within their jurisdictions, but with attached conditions regarding the ways in which the money was to be spent. For instance, it was during this period that the *Canada Assistance Plan* (1966) for social welfare, the *Hospital Insurance and Diagnostic Act* (1957) for hospital services, and the *Medical Care Act* (1966) for physician services, were all enacted at the federal level. These programs, by virtue of which the federal and provincial governments shared health-care costs equally, extended the policy capacity of the provincial government.

Far from being a period of unfettered state expansion at the expense of private interests, these years often saw the development of the service-delivery capacity of private practitioners (e.g. doctors), non-profit organizations (e.g. hospitals and community-based agencies), *and* private for-profit organizations. (OHHCPA, 2001; Mishra et al., 1988) The combination of public finance and private delivery has remained a hallmark of Ontario's health-care system. Although groups argued at the time that the expansion of the state into the realm of social and health service funding and delivery would create redundancies and reduce the need for non-profit organizations, others argued that the expansion of the state would allow these organizations to pursue more autonomous goals:

...[t]his spectacular growth in state welfare, far from super-seding the non-governmental organizations in fact helped in their proliferation. The secret of this relationship is that the government funded a variety of voluntary organizations, old and new, and entrusted many of them with the delivery of services. The growth of the government did not mean a de-cline of the non-governmental sector, indeed quite the oppo-site. Moreover, this post-war expansion of social-welfare ac-tivities also helped the development of the commercial sec-tor—profit-making organizations involved in the delivery of social welfare. (Mishra et al., 1988, 122)

Thus, the period extending from post-WWII until the mid-1970s was marked by a tremendous amount of state involvement in provid-ing grants and subsidies to both municipal institutions and charitable organizations to provide and extend the state's service-delivery capac-ity.

Formal State Program Funding for Home Care

The evolution of formal state involvement in funding and deliv-ering home-care services coincided with the expansion of the welfare state; however, it was a long time before consistent programs and serv-ices were available across the province. Both the Ministry of Commu-nity and Social Services (MCSS) and the Ministry of Health funded home-care programs. The province became formally involved with consistent programmatic funding of home care in 1958 with the in-troduction of the *Homemakers and Nurses Services Act*. Under the ae-gis of MCSS, this act enabled municipalities to hire nurses and home-makers directly, or to provide a contract to non-profit voluntary or-ganizations (e.g. Red Cross, Saint Elizabeth Visiting Nurses Associa-tion, the Victorian Order of Nurses). (Williams, 1996) It was during this period, with the growth in available funds and the identification of growing need, that non-profit organizations became fully fledged partners of the government. Individuals who received services under this program were charged according to their ability to pay, but the majority of the costs for the programs were shared on a fifty-fifty basis, with half covered jointly by the federal and provincial governments, and the other half funded by the municipality. The program administration was under the aegis of municipalities. By the late 1960s, the portion of the program that was financed by Ottawa and the provinces rose from fifty percent to eighty percent of the total cost. It was during this period that the program was extended to enable the provision of preventative care, respite care and emergency services. This program expansion led predictably to a large growth in demand. Further expansion of services resulted when amendments to the *Elderly Persons Social and Recreational Act, 1961*, made in 1966, enabled provincial funds to be directed towards non-profit voluntary organizations to provide home support services such as meals-on-wheels, home cleaning, shopping and other activities of daily living. (Williams, 1996) During this period, the Ministry of Community and Social Services was also actively engaged in funding other non-medical support services.

The Ontario Ministry of Health also began consistent funding of professional and paraprofessional services with the initiation of the Home Care Programs (HCPs) during the 1960s. In 1968, the *Acute Home Care Program* was introduced. The acute program was initially designed to provide medically oriented short-term professional health services (including nursing and rehabilitation services) to beneficiaries of the *Ontario Health Insurance Program* (OHIP). The intended outcome was rehabilitation for eligible recipients.

In 1974, the Ministry of Health created District Health Councils (DHCs) to plan and co-ordinate services regionally. The DHCs were able to contribute to the debate that was heating up over the lack of a home care "system." During this period, many DHCs conducted extensive studies that served to highlight the existing inadequacy of the links between the hospital and the community, as well as the lack of access to home care and community-care services. (Jenson & Phillips, 2000)

On the Path to Market: State Restructuring and Non-Profit Contractors (1971 - 2001)

By the mid-1970s, the advent of the first economic shocks since the large-scale expansion of the welfare state caused the more conservative elements within the ruling Conservative Party in Ontario to advocate policies of "retrenchment" and "restraint." Even before the dawn of Reaganism and Thatcherism, Ontario had already begun downsizing government significantly. (Mishra et al., 1988) A series of reports in the early 1970s supported restricting state growth. The Committee on Government Productivity (1969-1973) primarily focused on "...improvements in the structure and functioning of the government from the viewpoint of increasing efficiency and cutting costs." (Mishra et al. 1988, 153) Its report predicted that the 1970s would contrast with the optimistic 1960s, during which public spending had expanded. Decreased government revenues combined with increasing government obligations and commitments spelled a need for fiscal caution. While "privatization" of service delivery was advocated as a means to realize improved government efficiency and reduced spending, the report argued that policy-making should remain under the auspices of the state. The report also argued that the use of non-governmental organizations (non-profit, for-profit and voluntary) on a contract basis could provide a bulwark against increases in government spending. "Selective re-privatization of program delivery" could tap into the skills that were available at the community level, in non-profit organizations, in private for-profit organizations, or in community organizations sponsored by special-interest groups. (Committee on Government Productivity, 1971)

In line with the recommendations made in the Committee's report, the Budget of 1975 proposed limiting provincial spending growth and re-aligning state priorities with population needs. The Special Programme Review Committee (SPRC) reported during this period that an ever-expanding public purse was an "economic threat" to the future prosperity of Ontario. (Mishra et al., 1988) The SPRC called for reduced government growth and limits on spending. The report blamed the provincial budget deficit for boosting inflation, increasing interest rates, and reducing private investment in the province. It rejected the possibility of tackling the deficit by raising the tax rate, as higher taxes would constitute a direct disincentive to private investment, enterprise and productivity. (Ontario, 1975)

The SPRC's one-hundred and eighty-four recommendations heralded an overall shift in policy toward downsizing government and reducing social expenditures. But, more central to this analysis, these recommendations are critically important milestones in understanding the evolution of the relationship between the provincial government and voluntary non-profit organizations. These policies implemented a policy framework that favoured the withdrawal of the state from the delivery of services and elevated voluntary non-profit organizations from marginal players in the welfare state to full-fledged partners with government, delivering services on behalf of government and spotting opportunities to expand the reach of the public purse in the pursuit of social welfare goals.

Throughout this period, there was a growing sentiment both on the left and the right of the political spectrum that the state was not doing an adequate job in social welfare and that the welfare state was in crisis. (Rice & Prince, 2000) Out of the hum of discontent, the interests of two separate policy communities coalesced in the early 1980s around the processes of "debureaucratization" and "decentralization" of welfare state funding and service delivery. (Rekart, 1993; Mishra *et. al*, 1988) Neo-liberals calling for a decreased role for the state converged with advocates of welfare pluralism. Both groups hoped to reduce the influence of the state and to increase the capacity within communities. Both also advocated the increasing importance of voluntary community-based groups. Ironically, what neither group considered was the long-term implication of a withdrawal of the state. The neo-liberal policy community was united in its belief in curtailing direct government funding and delivery of health and social services. It argued that the state should merely reproduce the competitive conditions necessary for a market economy to flourish, while leaving other responsibilities to individuals, families, and mediating institutions, such as voluntary sector organizations.

The welfare-pluralist policy community was defined by its heterogeneous, grassroots nature. Its advocates increasingly called for the empowerment of community-based organizations. They also believed that grassroots organizations should be given the authority to promote the welfare of local communities. They criticized the failure of the welfare state to deliver on its promise to achieve equity and eradicate poverty. They also called for the decentralization of certain state services.

Both welfare pluralists and neo-liberals supported decentralization and active citizen engagement. (Mishra et al. 1988, Rekart, 1993) Welfare pluralists supported more voluntary-sector participation, but not necessarily less government. Although advocating a lesser role for the state, welfare pluralists pointed out that their project was not to be confused with the neo-liberal project of disengagement or minimal government. Yet, in spite of their quite different prescriptions, the voices of welfare pluralists inadvertently helped to support subsequent state retrenchment emerging from neo-liberal ideas.

In its submission to the Macdonald Commission (1984), the Canadian Association of Social Workers urged the commissioners to "consider voluntary organizations and associations of employers and employees as vehicles for the administration of social benefits. Community-based voluntary associations are a long-established tradition in Canada. They are non-profit in nature (and) (…) deliver a broad range of human services. They are capable of doing more." (Drover, 1983) Organizations such as the Social Planning Council of Metropolitan Toronto argued that the institutionalized welfare state did not alleviate the social ills of poverty, inequality and social need. Significant levels of poverty remained, while the growth of the tax-and-transfer system had not resulted in a more equitable distribution of income over a thirty-year period. Social programs were tainted by their stigmatizing elements, and the welfare state was perceived as bureaucratic, inflexible, and unresponsive to community needs. (Drache, Cameron & Social Planning Council of Metro Toronto, 1985) Scepticism regarding the state's ability to reduce inequalities led to renewed interest in the role of the voluntary sector. (Hadley & Hatch, 1981)

Throughout the 1980s, the ever greater influence of neo-liberal ideas on public policy altered the state's relationship to the market and the non-profit sector. As Tuohy aptly demonstrates in her analysis of the dynamics of health care in Canada, the United States and Britain, the "fiscal scope of the welfare state slowed in average in the 1980s, and public health was no exception to this phenomenon." More important than fiscal restraint, however, "was the development of a set of agendas for redesigning welfare-state programs and institutions." (1999: 3-4) In other words, the scaling back of the state took place in obvious ways with constraints to funding, but more subtly and insidiously with real shifts toward new agendas for state programs and institutions.

As Western nations began the process of creating these new agendas, they became more interested in non-governmental alternatives for the delivery of social services. Salamon uses the concept of "third-party government" to describe a pervasive trend for the federal government in the United States to shift the role of service provision to third parties, such as states, cities, and the non-profit sector. (Salamon, 1995) Wolch uses the concept of a "shadow state" to convey the idea that state restructuring in the United States involved a transfer of responsibilities from the public to the non-profit sector. (Wolch, 1990) Rekart traces the development of a new role for non-profit organizations as *public agents* in British Columbia during the 1960s and 1970s. (Rekart, 1993) Each of these analyses emphasizes that the non-profit sector remained financially dependent upon strong state support. This is a view shared by other observers. (Browne, 2000, 1996; Brooks, 1999; Hall & Reed, 1998; Mishra et al., 1988)

The government's reliance on voluntary non-profit organizations resulted in an elevated role for some organizations. The executive directors of voluntary non-profits were given access to government to influence policy, organizations were held up as archetypes of efficient and effective service delivery, and were called on to administer programs. Community support organizations increasingly tapped into available provincial, local and federal government funds to support locally developed home care programs and services for the elderly in their communities.

Towards a Home Care "System"

State commitment to implementing new home-care programs continued throughout the late 1970s and 1980s. By 1975, the Home Care Programs were extended to include care recipients requiring professional chronic care. The *Chronic Home Care Program* was first introduced on a pilot basis. It was gradually rolled out across the province, and was finally fully implemented in 1984 with the introduction of the Toronto program. Its primary objective was maintenance of health. As a result, care plans could last anywhere from months to years. (Williams, 1996) Many subsequent additions to the program extended the number of eligible individuals. The *School Health Program* (1984) provided services directly to eligible children in their schools. The *Integrated Homemaker Program* (1986) aimed to provide home and personal support services to recipients of professional home-care services. This program was funded by the Ministry of Community and Social Services (MCSS), but was administered locally through the Ministry of Health HCPs. Finally the *Assistive Devices Program* (1982) funded by the Ministry of Health contributed seventy-five percent of the purchase price of designated equipment for eligible clients.

In addition to the HCPs, two other programs were instituted. First, many government-funded non-profits were brought together under an umbrella organization called the *Home Support Program for the Elderly*. (Williams, 1996; Deber & Williams, 1995) Approximately 200 non-profit voluntary agencies joined. The range of services provided by these organizations included home support services such as wheels-to-meals, meals-on-wheels, friendly visiting, security checks, and transportation.

Secondly, the provincial government introduced a *Placement Coordination Service* (PCS). (Williams, 1996) The goal of this service was to act as a single point of access for care for recipients who needed long-term institutional care, community programs or a combination thereof. HCPs run alongside the PCS purchased nursing, homemaking, and other professional services on a contract basis from both for-profit and non-profit organizations. (Williams, 1996; Ontario Home Health Care Providers Association, 2001)

The Commodity of Care   81

By the late 1980s, home care in Ontario was maturing. As of 1989, there were thirty-eight locally administered HCPs operating across the province. In twenty-nine localities, local boards of health or public health units administered the HCPs. Three programs were administered by local hospitals, four by the Victorian Order of Nurses (VON), and a single program operated as a freestanding structure (Price Waterhouse, 1989).

Although much progress had been made, problems remained. Community support services were not available uniformly throughout the province. Nor were professional and para-professional services operating smoothly. In 1986, the provincial government initiated a reform of home care. Price Waterhouse, a private consulting firm, conducted a formal operational review of Ontario's home-care program on behalf of the provincial government. The review cited numerous problems. For example, it identified a conflict of interest in the fact that provider agencies, such as hospitals and the VON, were administering HCPs and thus determining both program eligibility and service delivery.[5] (Price Waterhouse, 1989) The report's authors warned that problems could arise when program administration and service delivery were joined in the same organization. They recommended that service providers not administer local programs. They also found that HCPs did not all operate in the same way. For instance, not all local programs used written service contracts with provider agencies. Among the programs that used contracts, quality assurance standards or guidelines were not always stipulated. A number of the consultants' recommendations made it into the home-care model eventually adopted by the province.

A series of reports prepared between 1986 and 1996 outlined several options for the provincial administration, regulation, and financing of home care. (Table 1)

Access to services (information about them and their delivery) was considered the biggest obstacle to a better system. The issue was confusing by virtue of the many levels of government involved, the many agencies providing different kinds of services, and schemes under which some services were free, while others might require payment of a user fee, depending on who referred the client to the home-

82 Canadian Centre for Policy Alternatives

Table 1 Proposed Long-Term-Care Reform Models (1986 - 1996)			
Governing Party	**Report Title**	**Home Care Access Model**	**Date of Report**
Liberal Party	New Agenda	One-Stop Shopping	1986
	Strategies for Change	Service Access Organizations	1990
New Democratic Party	Redirection of Long-Term Care and Support Services in Ontario	Service Coordination Agencies	1991
	Partnerships in Long-Term Care (4 reports)	Multi-Service Agencies	1993
Progressive Conservative Party	Alternatives to the MSA	Community Care Access Centres	1996

Source: Daly, 2003, 102

care agency. In large part, the reform process was driven by consumer demands for a simpler way of obtaining and arranging services. Simplifying access was therefore the chief goal of all of the reports listed in Table 1.

Throughout the 1980s and the first half of the 1990s, Ontario's Liberal, NDP and Conservative governments grappled with the various reform models, which "varied in the degree of involvement by the public and private sectors, in the financing and delivery of [home care] services, and in how these models can be represented along the continuum from centrally planned to market models." (Baranek et al., 1999) Each of the governments "put its distinctive stamp on reform proposals, consistent with its philosophy of the role of the state relative to the other two sectors." (Jenson & Phillips, 2000) Reforms to the administration, regulation and funding of home care were implemented incrementally throughout the reform period. (Daly, 2003) However, the key reform, creation of a single point of access for home and long-term care services, eluded full implementation until Mike Harris's government was able to push through its preferred model of managed competition in 1996. Community support services were left out of the final reform model. (Baranek, 2000; Baranek et al., 1999)

During the early 1990s, the administration of home care, which had been divided between the MCSS and the Ministry of Health was consolidated within the latter. Acute and chronic care in the home had been insured under the Ontario Health Insurance Plan (OHIP). Homemaking and community support services had been paid for by the Integrated Homemaker Program of the Ministry of Community and Social Services. In 1992, local community support organizations were transferred from the funding authority of the Ministry of Community and Social Services (MCSS) to that of the amalgamated Ministry of Health and Long Term Care (MOHLTC). In 1994, a single funding envelope for both categories of service was established within the MOHLTC, in essence creating a fixed annual budget for home-care services.

Under MCSS, the province had funded non-profit organizations or municipalities to provide community support services based on funding proposals. Regulatory restrictions attached to the Canada Assistance Plan (CAP), under which the MCSS received a large proportion of its funding, favoured the use of non-profit organizations. (Mishra et al., 1988) Once the federal government had cut its transfer to Ontario by imposing its "cap on CAP," there was little incentive to maintain home care under the aegis of the MCSS, which had until then seen the federal government share half of the cost of its home-care programs.[6] Unlike the MCSS, the MOHLTC harboured no commitment to fund non-profit organizations to deliver services, rather than for-profit businesses. However, in 1995, when the Harris government came to power, para-professional and professional home-care services were still primarily delivered (and sometimes administered) by non-profits such as the Victorian Order of Nurses and the Red Cross, despite in-roads made by for-profit organizations. (OACCAC, 2001) The dominance of non-profit organizations in home-care service provision did not end until the introduction of market-based reforms and the initiation of full competition for service contracts in 1996. Ontario's regionally based managed-competition model for professional and paraprofessional home-care services entrenched a competitive process for the awarding of contracts, opening competitions to both non-profit and for-profit providers through the use of a "request-for-proposal" process. Competition for contracts to provide extended health care does not contravene the Canada Health Act (CHA).[7] The latter does not enable the federal government to restrict provinces from using for-profit providers to deliver extended health-care services (e.g. home-care services). (Hollander et al, 2000) Nevertheless, the decision to create a competitive brokerage model for home-care services and to fund community support non-profit organiza-

84   Canadian Centre for Policy Alternatives

tions on a quasi-fee-for-service basis challenges the relationships that existed between non-profit organizations and the state during the period before 1996.

3. The Contours of State Retrenchment in Home Care

Recall that *programmatic retrenchment* may involve cutting expenditures, instituting more or different rules and regulations in the design of programs, and making programs merely residual (Rice & Prince, 2000; Pierson, 1994) The provincial government's commitment to fund *some* home-care services remains high, while some others have suffered from programmatic retrenchment. Overall funding has increased, but has not kept up with the demand for some services, while other services have seen substantial cuts. Funding for some community support services has more grown more rapidly than for others. The rules governing professional and paraprofessional non-profit organizations have become more idiosyncratic since the implementation of managed competition. The reporting requirements for community-support non-profit organizations have become increasingly strict and rigid.

Changes to Rules and Regulations

The home-care budget is presently divided into two parts.[8] One flows through the province's forty-three Community Care Access Centres (CCACs). The legislation creating the CCACs was enacted in 1996 as an amendment of the *Long Term Care Act*. The CCACs became active in 1997, officially operating as non-governmental, non-profit organizations (some CCACs have also recently become registered charities). Responsibility for administration and allocation of publicly funded professional and paraprofessional home-care services shifted from the province to CCACs. The latter's mandate includes case management, referrals to day programs, and placement in long-term care institutions. In some communities, though not all, CCACs are a major source of referrals to community support programs. However, CCACs are not permitted to provide any other direct services. They award contracts for professional (nursing and rehabilitation services) and paraprofessional services (personal support work/homemaking) to for-profit and non-profit organizations that successfully bid for them in response to requests for proposals.

In many instances, CCACs stipulate the type of information that provider agencies must report. CCACs use this information for planning and evaluation purposes. Each of the forty-three CCACs currently requires the provider agencies to submit different information for the RFP process and for contract-compliance monitoring. This complicates matters for agencies that have contracts with several CCACs. In addition, due to the competitive nature of the home-care market, the data collected from provider agencies is not publicly available. Each CCAC reports aggregate statistics differently in its annual report. This hinders adequate scrutiny, comparison, and public accountability.

The other part of the provincial home-care budget flows directly from the MOHLTC to community support organizations—both voluntary and local government-run—to provide a pre-defined basket of community support services, including home care (e.g. home help/homemaking, meals-on-wheels, security checks, transportation and friendly visiting). Organizations have a direct reporting relationship with regional MOHLTC program consultants. As of 1995, the MOHLTC instituted the *Planning, Funding and Accountability Policies and Procedures Manual for Long Term Care Services* (PFA). This manual represents a departure from how community support services were previously funded. The unconditional grants—or global funding—that organizations providing community support services received from the provincial government were replaced by "quasi" fee-for-service contracts. Mishra argues that "[w]ith the replacement of general unconditional grants with fee-for-service contracts [voluntary agencies] are in danger of becoming mere service providers, sometimes little more than contractors serving a particular department or ministry." (Mishra et al., 1988)

The original 1995 edition of the manual provided community support organizations with information on government priority-setting, budget processes, the community equity funding envelope, and the roles and responsibilities of the MOHLTC, district health councils, and the providers of community-support services. Subsequent revisions to this manual update the *service agreement* process (see below), planning, budgeting and reporting procedures, and stipulate any changes to MOHLTC policy affecting the delivery of long-term-care services. Once collected, funding and service statistics become part of the Community and Social Services database (CSS).

The contract between the MOHLTC and community support programs for direct funding is in two parts: a *Legal Agreement* outlines the organization's obligations and the annual *Service Agreement* stipulates the number of services that will be provided—in each category of funded MOHLTC services—to produce the line-by-line budget figures. Budgets (service agreements) are negotiated annually by the organizations with their regionally appointed MOHLTC program consultant. Budgets are based on two things: the total units of service that will be provided (measured in hours, visits, one-way trips, matches or meals) and the historical provincial funding allotted to the organization (primarily based on the previous year's funding). Funding allocations are made to organizations on a line-by-line basis—in what amounts to a quasi-fee-for-service payment—to provide the agreed-upon units of service. This is *quasi*-fee-for-service funding, since there is not a direct connection between the budget and the projected units of service. The historical amount of funding from the province—as a proportion of the organizations' total revenue—seems to be a determining factor in future budget allocations. Furthermore, although community-support organizations are expected to provide the agreed-upon units of service, they are not normally required to return money if they fail to meet their projections, as long as there is an adequate reason for the discrepancy.

Interviewees noted that the budget process is much more time-consuming than in the past, with each approved budget line requiring a narrative justification. In addition, budget lines cannot be easily moved around. There are opportunities for windfall funding, in the form of enhancement and expansion budgets. However, additional funding is more variable and requires a separate proposal. It is also contingent upon the availability of funds. Organizations are only funded to provide the "basket of services." They are required to maintain levels of fundraising and user fees but are not supposed to use Ministry-funded staff time for these tasks. In this sector, few organizations are large enough to have a fundraising machinery. They note that it is difficult to motivate boards to engage in fundraising. Given the inflexibility of their funding, organizations are making choices about how to continue to provide services, especially to groups at risk such as the frail elderly. Some organizations have decreased their hours of operation to cope with shortfalls.

Funding for Home-Care Services

There are at least four discernable trends in the way public funding of home care has been altered by managed competition. First, overall funding has increased, but not in keeping with demand. At first glance, it does not appear that there has been fiscal restraint in the home-care sector. Coyte, Hall and Croxford (1999) point out that public-sector funding for home care in all of Canada has increased dramatically in the last two decades, rising from $62.3 million in 1975/ 76 to $2,096.0 million in 1996/97. This increase represents an average annual rate of growth of just over seventeen percent which is more than triple the general rate of inflation (5.3%) over the same period. However, these expenditures still account for less than four percent of all public-sector spending on health care in Canada. In Ontario, the average annual growth rate of almost 19 percent for home care exceeded the annual growth rate of just over 17 percent for Canada as a whole. Ontario's per capita spending of $91.08 in 1996/97 also exceeded the $69.20 per capita home care rate for all of Canada (Coyte, Hall & Croxford, 1999).

Browne (2000) notes that Ontario provincial government expenditures on home care services (in constant 2000 dollars) have grown from $ 1,089,363,739 in 1994/95 to an estimated $ 1,521,766,419 in fiscal 2000/01. This represents an average annual growth rate of just under six percent. Overall growth for the period between 1995/ 96 and 2000/01 for *all* services in the home-care envelope—including both professional and homemaking/personal-support services, personal support/attendant outreach, supportive housing, acquired brain injury, children's treatment centres, and community-support services—was 36.4 percent (Table 2). By way of comparison, the overall growth for all health care spending for the same time period in Ontario in 2000 constant dollars was 13.4 percent. Given that the growth in home-care expenditures far exceeds the growth of health-care spending as a whole, is it legitimate to claim that state retrenchment is occurring in this sector? Yes, if we look at the budgets for individual services: the state is changing which services it funds.

The growth rate for individual home-care services varied considerably over the period under review. Community-support and professional home-care services (at rates of 34 and 32 percent respectively) did not grow as quickly as overall expenditure. Homemaking grew most rapidly with a 47 percent increase. Based on these figures, it is clear that not all home-care services have grown equally.

Although the annual average growth rate for community support services between 1995/96 and 2000/2001 was 7 percent, there was wide variation here too between individual services (Table 3). Without detracting from the concerns of associations such as the Ontario Community Support Association and the Ontario Home Health Care Providers Association regarding turmoil in professional and paraprofessional home-care services, expenditures for others community support services such as diners' club and home help/homemaking haved declined by 44.4 percent and 43.8 percent respectively in the past five years. Since all health- and-social-care services are funded from the same envelope, an implicit competition between various services exists. In other words, funding growth in one service is counterbalanced by lower growth in another.

Third, funding growth may mask problems associated with a higher demand for services. Browne notes that between 1996/97 and 1998/99 homemaking hours purchased by CCACs increased by nearly 25 percent, less than the 30 percent growth in the number of profes-

Table 2 Total Growth, 1995/96 to 2000/01	
Expenditure Growth for Selected Home Care Service & Growth for Overall Expenditures for all Home Care Services	**Percentage Growth in Expenditures**
Community Support	34%
Professional Services	32%
Homemaking/ Personal Support Work	47%
Overall Growth (All Services)	36%

Analysis based on figures from Browne (2000, 90)

The Commodity of Care   89

Table 3
Growth Rates for Community-Support Services
All of Ontario, 1995/1996 to 2000/2001
(1992 Constant Dollars)

	Overall Growth Rates
Adult Day Services (01A, 01B, 01C, 01D)	56%
Meals on Wheels (02A)	17.4%
Diners' Club/Wheels to Meals/Congregate Dining (03A	-44.4%
Transportation (04A)	51.5%
Home Maintenance and Repair (05A + 05C)	27.7%
Friendly Visiting (06A)	50.3%
Security Checks or Reassurance Services (07A)	19.4%
Caregiver Support (08A)	27.0%
Home Help/Homemaking (09B, 09P)	-43.8%
Intervention and Assistance Services (Seniors) (09I)	0.04%

Source: Daly (2003, 182)

Table 4
Day Procedures by Selected District Health Council, Region of Facility Location, Compared
with All DHC Regions in Ontario and all Regions in Canada

Selected District Health Council (DHC) Regions, All DHCs in Ontario & All Regions in Canada	1994-95	1995-96	1996-97	1997-98	1998-99
Waterloo Wellington Dufferin DHC	16.3%	6.1%	4.6%	2.0%	0.5%
Toronto	3.3%	5.6%	3.3%	(2.5%)	4.0%
Halton-Peel District Health Council	63.5%	5.0%	8.3%	2.2%	22.5%
Hamilton-Wentworth DHC	(31.7%)	5.2%	3.4%	2.3%	5.0%
Ontario	3.2%	3.5%	7.1%	1.4%	4.7%
Canada	6.7%	(8.2%)	(2.8%)	2.9%	4.4%

Source: (CIHI) Canadian Institute for Health Information http://secure.cihi.ca (2002). *Day Procedures by Region of Facility Location*. Accessed August, 2002.

sional service visits that were purchased. But these figures have not been correlated with changes in demand. Interviewees pointed out that with hospital restructuring, both decreases made to lengths of stay and the increasing number of day procedures performed have combined to put pressure on demand for CCAC and community support services. In all regions, day procedure rates have increased and in some such as Halton-Peel they have increased year over year (Table 4).

Other factors have also driven the rising demand for services. Community support organizations are facing an increased demand for their services from individuals referred to them by CCACs, or not served by the CCAC, but especially from individuals on CCAC waiting lists. Clients require more care due to a higher level of acuity.

They are also continuing to live in their homes, rather than moving to institutions. Despite demand, some community support services have grown while others have experienced overall decline.

Fourth, funding constraints imposed in June 2001 had a tremendous impact on the availability of service. Despite the large growth of 47 percent in the homemaking/personal support work category for the years between 1995/96 and 2000/01, interviewees report that homemaking services (e.g. cleaning, meal preparation, laundry) were cut tremendously when CCAC funding cutbacks began in June 2001. Prior to the June 2001 funding cap, the MOHLTC either increased CCACs' budgets to meet the growth in demand for services or CCACs received deficit financing. In June 2001, when the MOHLTC announced that it would discontinue its practice of covering CCAC deficits, CCACs were told to hold service levels constant. For some CCACs, such as Wellington-Dufferin, that had been operating within their funding envelope, the freeze had a less drastic, immediate impact. Others, such as Waterloo Region CCAC, which had been operating on the basis of client demand, were forced to implement expenditure controls immediately. Province-wide, CCACs were faced with a collective projected deficit of $175 million in fiscal 2001/02. (Community Care Access Centre of Waterloo Region 2001b)

A survey conducted by the Ontario Association of Community Care Access Centres, and reported by Waterloo CCAC to its Board of Directors, indicated that CCACs were adopting a variety of measures to cope with the reduction in funding, including, but not limited to, the following:

- implement waiting lists;
- prioritizing clients;
- eliminating clients on waiting lists or receiving services from another community organization or institution;
- reducing or eliminating medical supplies;
- eliminating services to clients who are ambulatory or otherwise mobile;
- increasing case management assessments;
- reducing or eliminating components of clinical service;
- reducing internal CCAC staff;

- freezing program development and capital expenditures; and
- making operational and administrative reductions. (Community Care Access Centre of Waterloo Region 2001b)

In response to the requirement to reduce expenditures, the Waterloo CCAC developed a cost-containment strategy, consisting in:

- the establishment of waiting lists for homemaking services, enterostomal therapy/wound management, and Alzheimer Respite;
- the restriction of CCAC admissions to those individuals able to access outpatient services;
- the creation of quotas for referrals for nursing services, combined with a lowering of the ceilings for nursing services and a review of CCAC services provided to individuals in retirement homes. (Marosi 2001)

With expenditure controls in place clients receive fewer hours of personal care on average.

…when we implemented the expenditure controls, we were managing to a budget. We were not managing in any way to client need. I mean there was full acknowledgement of that, that in terms of what clients were being assessed as requiring, they were not receiving it. And we were not allocating—we went from an average of 22 hours of personal care a month, to today around 14 hours. And you know, [we] went from a client case load of around 7,000 to 6,500, so to argue in any way that those 500 people that were on the case load didn't need the services would just not be valid. I mean they were assessed by professionals as needing the services and…the bar has been raised now. People have to be sicker to get the services. And they have to be much sicker to get the same level of service that they were getting before. So…it really would be erroneous to pretend that…there was an exact science that went into place…in terms of the determination…of the reductions, and which reductions would be made, these were seen as the reductions that in the whole continuum of what we provide would have the least impact. But it was acknowl-

92   Canadian Centre for Policy Alternatives

edged that it was a very serious, negative impact. (Interview 051402)

The CCAC noted that it had to "severely constrain" the number of clients admitted for homemaking and personal support services following expenditure controls. During the case-management assessment, clients were screened according to priority on the basis of disability stratification, living arrangements, burden assessment and length of wait (A,B,C and D). Since the June 2001 implementation of expenditure controls, "A" clients were admitted for service, while "B" and "C" clients were put onto waiting lists. (Table 5). The CCAC switched the proportions of admissions to discharges from 1:8 in May 2001 to 1:1 by December 2001. By December, the waiting lists for homemaking/personal support started to decline, as clients were admitted to service, or pursued other alternatives. Between June and December 2001, 276 clients were admitted from the "B' and "C" lists, and 294 clients were discharged without receiving service. Of clients who declined services (more than 60), 20 percent indicated that their family would provide the care, while 23 percent preferred to purchase services privately. Of those discharged from the waiting list due to institutionalization (more than 80 clients), 61 percent were hospitalized (meaning they were sick enough to enter hospital), 27 percent were transferred to long-term-care facilities, and 12 percent went into retirement homes. (Community Care Access Centre of Waterloo Region 2002)

The CCAC also indicated that referrals for nursing care steadily declined as a result of expenditure control as services for some ambulatory clients were eliminated. In 2001, the overall caseload for nursing was significantly lower than the previous year, due to a lower number of referrals from hospitals overall and to nursing shortages.

Table 5 Snapshot of Waiting Lists at Two Points in Time		
Priority Code	October 31, 2001	January 7, 2002
A	0	0
B	152	16
C	197	127
D	293	356

Source: (Community Care Access Centre of Waterloo Region 2002)

A study of Waterloo Region CCAC clients concluded that recipients of homemaking/ personal support work tended to be "older, female, widowed, living alone, less able to get out of the home, more disabled, more cognitively impaired, longer-term clients and at higher risk of institutionalization compared with non-recipients." (Hirdes, Dalby et. al, 2001) The vulnerability of the clients receiving personal support poses potential consequences for decisions to restrict access to these services.

To conclude: the rules and reporting requirements for professional and paraprofessional provider organizations, non-profit and for-profit alike, have increased and become more idiosyncratic, reflecting a lack of coherent direction from the state. The reporting and budgeting requirements for community support non-profits have also become more complex and burdensome. The state has both expanded and cut back its funding of home care. Overall, levels of funding have increased. However, some services are no longer offered in sufficient quantity to meet demand. This has placed an increased burden on family, friends, and voluntary organizations to assume responsibility for the care of those in need.

4. Emerging Issues: Managing At the Margins?

Capacity for Competitiveness

The Ontario government signed an increasing number of contracts with for-profit commercial organizations for professional and paraprofessional services between 1974 and the mid-1980s. In Metropolitan Toronto, for example, the number of for-profit organizations with contracts to deliver home-care services *tripled* between 1974 and 1984. (Mishra *et al.*, 1988) By 1983/84, at least half of the Ministry of Health's $18 million dollars' worth of Home-Care-Program contracts were with for-profit organizations. (Mishra et al. 1988) The use of for-profit providers in Waterloo region dates back to the early 1980s. According to the Ontario Home Health Care Providers Association private for-profit organizations have delivered home-care services for the past thirty years in Ontario. (OHHCPA, 2001) For-profits held shift nursing, overflow and weekend nursing duty contracts with local Home Care Programs. Even before the introduction of the managed-competition model for home-care services in 1996, the role of the for-profit sector in the delivery of health-related home-care services was growing. (Mishra et al., 1988)

While for-profit businesses may have held an increasing number of contracts, non-profit organizations still retained more than 60 percent of the hours and 80 percent of the visits for nursing in 1995. However, by 2000, the ratios had changed to just over 40 percent of the hours and less than 60 percent of the visits (see Figures 2 and 3). (OACCAC, 2001) The percentage of *nursing* hours and visits performed by professional and paraprofessional non-profit organizations has predictably declined. Initial results from a survey of 41 of 43 CCACs conducted by the Ontario Association for Community Care Access Centres (OACCAC) reveals that the percentage of contracted visits done by registered nurses with non-profit organizations declined by nearly 30 percentage points between 1995 and 2000 from 89 percent to 60 percent (see Figure 2). The share of registered practical nursing (RPN) visits also diminished by just under 25 percentage

Figure 2
Contracted Visits by RNs and RPNs, 1995 and 2000

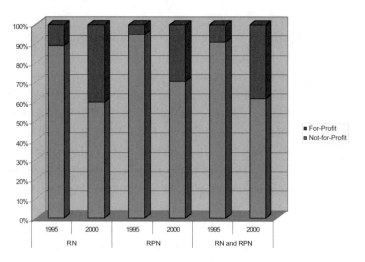

Source: Ontario Association of Community Care Access Centres, 2001

Figure 3
Hours of Contracted Work by RNs and RPNs, For-profit and Not-for-profit Organizations, 1995 and 2000

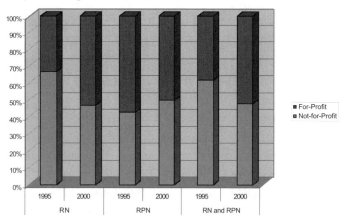

Source: Ontario Association of Community Care Access Centres, 2001

points for non-profit organizations, from 95 percent to 71 percent over the same period.[9] (OACCAC, 2001)

Non-profit organizations have lost a lot of ground when it comes to nursing and RPN *visits* (as was expected). However, their share of nursing *hours* has decreased less (20 percentage points) than the decrease in the number of visits (29 percentage points). Meanwhile, their share of RPN *hours* has increased (7 percentage points), while their share of RPN *visits* has declined (24 percentage points), reflecting a higher level of acuity among clients. Although the data are useful to show the aggregate market share of for-profit compared with non-profit nursing and RPN providers in the period before and after the introduction of the RFP, the data do not in themselves explain the differences, if any, between the ways that private for-profit and non-profit organizations provide professional and paraprofessional services. This issue is further complicated by the fact that information sharing has been reduced since the implementation of the RFP, as information is increasingly a proprietary commodity in establishing or maintaining market control.

While for-profits may have provided certain types of professional and paraprofessional services in the past, this was generally restricted to services that the main non-profit organization was unable to deliver. In other words, for-profits typically provided services when the non-profits were unable to do so. In the current environment, for-profits are able to compete more fully for service contracts. As a result, professional and paraprofessional non-profit organizations have had to act more like competitive businesses in order to win contracts. This has worked well in some cases where non-profits have expanded into new territories. It has also had a devastating impact on other non-profits.

The Red Cross just recently lost a contract with *Durham Access to Care*, reversing a 43-year long relationship with that community. (Soo, 2001) The VON has experienced similar difficulties in a number of communities, notably in Wellington-Dufferin in February 2002, where its local branch was ruled ineligible to bid in the RFP, because it was heavily in debt. (Kelly, 2002) The branch has since closed its operations entirely after serving the regions of Waterloo and Wellington-Dufferin for over ninety years. The decision followed the loss of a nursing contract in February 2002, and the subsequent loss of personal support/homemaking in Wellington-Dufferin and for nursing in Waterloo. The Wellington-Dufferin CCAC dropped the VON in the pre-qualification round of bidding for a new two-year nursing contract because the local VON branch was running a deficit. With an annual budget of $10.5 million, it ended the fiscal year in March 2001 with a deficit of $806,000, up from a deficit of $546,000 in 2000. (Kelly, 2002) New contracts were awarded to Saint-Elizabeth Health Care (a non-profit) and Care Partners. (Wellington-Dufferin CCAC 2002) The Wellington-Dufferin homemaking/personal-support contract was lost by VON in 2003, and awarded to Red Cross, HLO and Paramed. The nursing contract for Waterloo was lost in the 2003 RFP round, and services for Paramed, Comcare and Care Partners were expanded. In February 2003, the MOHLTC approved the transfer of all of the Waterloo & Wellington-Dufferin VON community support services (day-away program, meals on wheels, security checks, friendly visiting, and transportation) to the VON Peel Region Branch. (VON Canada 2003) Issues related to the impact of pay equity on the VON's full-time hourly paid nursing staff, and the debt acquired from merging two branches into one were cited as some of the reasons for its difficulties. (Interview 041702B; Interview 051402B; Interview 051602)

Both the Red Cross and the VON favoured decentralized branches, but experience with the RFP process has caused some re-thinking. Both organizations are now re-organizing, moving toward a more centralized, joint-head-office-and-local-branch structure. (Interview 062002; Interview 041702B)

Although provincial funding for CCAC home-care services has increased (and subsequently been capped) some organizations venture that it is the process of CCAC contract funding and the uncertainty of winning contracts through the submission of an RFP that has de-stabilized them. Mounting a bid in response to an RFP carries a high development price tag—at least $10,000 to $50,000 per proposal, according to informants. Just to be able to participate in the RFP process means that an organization has to be able to put together a competitive RFP, which requires tremendous amounts of administrative time and resources. In fact, if an organization is small, the RFP process seems to work against it, regardless of its for-profit or non-profit status. In response to the rigorous demands of the RFP, some organizations have been forced to merge or to form joint partnerships, consortiums, or formal legal corporations. New partnerships or consortiums have enabled some non-profit organizations to link with each other to provide professional and paraprofessional health services, or to expand their capacity across the province. More than one interviewee commented that competition has actually forced the quality of care to improve in all organizations regardless of their non-profit or for-profit status. (Interview 092801; Interview 043001A; Interview 043001B). But the interviewees were also quick to point out that the variety of request-for-proposal processes that are used across the province have created difficulties for organizations operating in more than one CCAC region. Decentralized or small organizations note that they lack the capacity at the branch level to deal with the rigorous demands of the RFP. Losing a contract for personal support work or nursing services, which can conservatively comprise anywhere from five percent to twenty-five percent of a non-profit service organization's budget, can be catastrophic for an organization, since the proceeds from contract work often go to support other social support services. (Interview 092801; Interview 043001A; Interview 050401)

The contracting process has caused staff attrition. When an organization loses a contract, interviewees report that their employees do not tend to go to work for other community agencies, but rather seek employment either in the institutional sector where wages are higher, or outside of the field. The ability to attract skilled human resources is a key criterion in remaining competitive. Competition based on price is therefore an issue for non-profits, since they are more likely to be unionized and thus pay higher wages to their personal-support workers.

While the news media has openly exposed the plight of branches of the Victorian Order of Nurses and the Red Cross Homemakers, Saint-Elizabeth Health Care has responded favourably to this new environment. What types of characteristics make it easier for some non-profit organizations to manage in this changed environment? The relationship between for-profit firms and non-profit organizations has shifted substantially since the introduction of managed competition: some interviewees stated that since the introduction of managed competition many organizations have been forced to act more as though they are businesses. Many are looking for other sources of revenue to survive contract loss. In some cases they have tried to generate revenue by offering new commercial services. (Tindale & MacLachlan, 2001)

Non-profits with professional or paraprofessional staff seem more likely to engage in commercial activities to fuel their organizational missions. Some organizations have been more successful than others. Many find that it is increasingly difficult to cope internally with two separate organizational cultures, a competitive market culture and an altruistic, voluntary one. One interviewee summed it up this way:

> ...[T]he community agencies are competing with special purpose organizations, in a sense. When the for-profits come into this business in a much larger way, you don't find a for-profit out there that also runs congregated dining, friendly visiting,

does crisis intervention, nor do they do home care. They send nurses out, and physiotherapists and homemakers. The other organizations have huge volunteer coordination challenges, all these other important and absolutely critical issues to manage, and home care is not their full focus, and yet they've got to compete on a contract with that, and so it drives their attention and their focus to the home-care side of things only, and so the resulting partnership agreements and all sorts of things are survival tactics to keep the organization alive and well, in order to be able to provide these other services. (Interview 010902)

While seeking new programmatic opportunities, VON branches studied by Tindale & MacLachlan (2001) indicated that they were hampered by a lack of resources for the extensive marketing needed to generate new business. The branches also note that they lack expertise in this area and are limited in their ability to hire consultants. Staff members of non-profit organizations are not always comfortable engaging in for-profit business ventures because they view themselves through the lens of a charitable organization. The cultural challenge is in "thinking like a business, and adopting marketing strategies." Sandra Hamner, formerly of Waterloo & Wellington-Dufferin VON, described her branch as a "charity run like a business." (Tindale and MacLachlan, 2001, 205-206)

For small, local community-support nonprofits, the focus is not on commercialization, but on the adoption of business-like management models and increasing the skills of their administrative staff, in part because government reporting requirements place an onus on them to do so. In order to understand the magnitude of this issue for very small informal organizations, one must recognize that some organizations still submit their budgets to the Ministry written in pencil and added by hand. (Interview 051502) Some organizations have only just acquired their first personal computer. Many lack e-mail, although most now have fax machines. In some cases, the Executive Director sorts the mail, assesses the clients, mixes with local politicians, coordinates the volunteers and stuffs envelopes. When it comes to dealing with the administrative requirements, such small, client focused organizations can be overwhelmed. Moreover, non-profits typically pay low salaries, making it difficult to attract new people who already have management experience and training.

Many of the larger community support non-profits report implementing new management techniques. They have marketing campaigns and brand imaging. They are using data systems to track their services. They try to attract corporate sponsorship. They are spending more time engaging in fundraising in order to stabilize their budgets, despite being restricted from fundraising on Ministry time. The fundraising they do needs to be more sophisticated as the field of competition grows. Opportunities to run charitable casinos are diminished as a result of the province's casinos. Bingos do not generate enough revenue, and pools of corporate donations are more difficult to access. (Interview 040202) In addition, the budget process is time intensive. Organizations report that it does not integrate well with their other organizational planning, or with other reporting requirements. The government also stipulates that historical levels of fundraising and user fees generated by an organization need to be maintained, as Ministry funding will not make up any shortfalls in these areas. The need to adopt business-like management models, as a result of the reporting requirements implemented with the reforms, make it difficult for very small organizations, lacking administrative expertise and human resources, to continue to operate. In some cases, small organizations with long histories have been absorbed by larger organizations, where the Ministry has deemed that their services are still needed in a community. (Interview 040202; Interview 051502) In other cases, organizations have ceased to exist. (Interview 011402)

Although there are distinctions between professional/paraprofessional non-profit organizations and the agencies that provide community support services depending on their level of involvement in the RFP, competition has blurred the boundaries between them. Professional and paraprofessional non-profits have made inroads into community support services in some areas, in part because of their overall lack of success in the RFP process.

In smaller communities, agencies such as the VON are providing more and more community support services formerly provided by small, local grassroots organizations. While many non-profits that were primarily involved in community support in Toronto also had contracts with the HCPs, they encountered difficulty with the move to the RFP process. In the initial rounds of contracting, CCACs reserved a certain percentage of contracted services for the non-profit organization(s) that had historically provided them. This exemption ended in 1999. Large, well-established non-profit organizations have lost significant contracts in some areas, while new "consortiums" of non-profits have emerged as competitors, notably within the six Toronto CCACs. For instance, Woodgreen and Senior Link have partnered to put in an RFP. Community-support-service agencies have also linked up.

This formal organizational cooperation represents a departure from the past. Prior to the implementation of the CCACs, organizations often worked together through informal networks, or through more formalized service partnerships. For example, one organization would provide a particular basket of services that complemented another organization's services, by coordinating geographic boundaries, hours of operation, or types of services. Since the creation of CCACs, organizations are not dismissing the idea of merging or continuing to amalgamate services on a more formalized basis. Indeed many organizations have submitted, or are planning to submit, RFPs together (as mentioned above) to help defray their costs and to improve their chances of success.

Efficiency and Accountability Without Autonomy

The culture of efficiency and accountability that has emerged as a major aspect of governing parallels the shift in the role of the state as contractor, regulator and partner. (Stein, 2001) This shift has impacted the relationship between the state and non-profit organizations.

The new role of the state as contractor, regulator, and partner should make it both easier and more difficult for states to meet at least some of these demands for accountability. The state as contractor and regulator now has no choice when it enters into contracts but to specify, in advance and with some precision, exactly what kinds of services are expected and what kinds of standards must be met. This is the hard part, for governments often do not have this kind of comprehensive information about the quality of public goods and the efficiency with which they are delivered. (Stein, 2001, 78)

In the home-care sector in Ontario, the MOHLTC uses the *Planning, Funding and Accountability* (PFA) manual to impose accountability or contract compliance on the community support programs that deliver services directly, and on CCACs that contract for professional and paraprofessional services. The MOHLTC monitors both community support programs (transfer payment agencies) and CCACs using service statistics submitted with the annual budgeting process and outlined in the PFA.

This new emphasis on accountability affects both community support programs and professional and paraprofessional agencies—but in different ways. Here I focus on issues emerging as a result of the *way* in which accountability is enforced by the state. Professional and para-professional non-profit organizations, like their for-profit counterparts, are accountable to individual CCACs and their boards. Information about the conduct of individual contractors is not normally a part of the CCAC public reporting. The public must trust that CCACs are ensuring the accountability of their contractors. The annual reports of the contractors are typically aggregated at too high a level for any meaningful local data to be revealed. By contrast, much more information exists about individual community support programs.

Community support programs are subject to the same accountability procedures as CCACs. Consequently, the administrative requirements on small community support agencies are sometimes burdensome, particularly if the organizations lack sufficient staff, computer systems to track information, or the time to do so properly. Interviewees routinely noted that funding from the provincial government for their base budget is very restrictive. Accountability requirements have caused organizations to shift their focus from client service to internal management. Unique local programs are no longer funded if they fall outside the PFA basket of services. This is a departure from the organizations' past autonomy, when "we wrapped our services around people not people around services." (Interview 051402A) Efficiencies can be gained with larger, multi-service organizations, where the added costs of administering programs can be borne throughout the organization. Smaller, stand-alone community support programs—akin to local "mom and pop shops"—cannot spread their administrative and overhead costs in quite the same way.

Organizations noted that the service data submitted to the Ministry as part of the PFA requirements are not reliable in the aggregate as a result of several data gathering problems.[10] The problems are primarily a function of the wide variation in the way organizations "count" units of service. There seems to be some recognition at a Ministry level that the data are not reliable, as program consultants typically use an organization's own historic service data to compare performance, year over year. But non-profit organizations point out that provincial "averages" for each service are circulated and used as benchmarks by program consultants. The MOHLTC expects organizations to operate as close to the "cost per unit of service average" as possible. But there are issues with this. The averages do not account for variation in counting units amongst different organizations, resulting in skewed averages, a problem that is well known in the community. Nor do the averages reflect the reality of rural non-profit organizations where travel and distance are pervasive issues. They argue that service-unit benchmarks do not reveal what they really accomplish. Key successes related to their organization's long-term social-welfare goals are difficult to measure quantitatively, and in any case are not collected by the Ministry. With the emphasis on accountability and outcomes, tied to breaking down every task into a unit of service (by hours, visits, matches or meals), and controlling precisely what types of services are eligible for MOHLTC funding, organizations feel that they lack the autonomy from government to focus on locally defined needs. They claim that they are forced to spend time figuring out how to "game" the system in order to accomplish the same social-welfare goals that the state openly supported in the past.

Local community support programs speak of a time when they used to have greater funding flexibility and more autonomy in the way that they could respond to local needs. In the past, they received core grants, which could be allocated flexibly within the organization. One interviewee remarked that the community-health sector had a tremendous amount of accountability under the old system, because of the need to report to boards of directors and to interact with local communities. Under the new model, base funding is very restricted; allocations are made to agencies on a line-by-line basis, for the delivery of specific services. In addition, budget lines cannot be easily moved around. Non-profit organizations argue that the government's accountability framework does not enable it to manage effectively.

Benchmarks—used as measures of efficiency—also do not account for the role small organizations play in promoting local community voluntary participation, a key ingredient of a healthy civil society and social cohesion. As efficient organizations, most non-profits leverage, on average, fifty volunteers for each full-time staff person. They indicate that they do not want to burden their volunteers, as it is already difficult to recruit them. They feel that this requires having a volunteer coordinator. Some organizations have them; many others, though, have not been able to convince the Ministry of the need, or have not had sufficient funds to warrant funding a new volunteer coordinator position. Without a full-time coordinator, or appropriate data systems in place to track services, the reporting requirements of the PFA can be difficult to manage. With most of their budget tied to the fees earned for performing contracted services, organizations feel that they cannot grow without more staff, but cannot get more staff unless they are providing much more service.

As the ideas of social cohesion are gaining ground as a "substitute" for the welfare state, the use of volunteers is being touted as a key expression of community. Government documents have been supporting the idea of increasing the use of volunteers for years. Politicians see non-profit organizations as repositories for volunteers to gain meaningful experiences. What politicians infrequently discuss is the cost to an organization that creates the benefits of social engagement and interaction for volunteers. Being a voluntary organization requires staff resources, opportunities, facilities, funding, and training resources. The costs of running good volunteer programs are often not recognized by the state; in government reports, volunteers are often treated as "free." The use of volunteers is being recommended by government. Yet, the policy tools governing the home-care sector reflect very little recognition of the amount of staff-time and money required to support voluntarism.

CCACs in the Home Care Continuum

Community care access centres now play a pivotal role in the home-care sector. Unfortunately, according to the interviews I conducted and to an Ontario Community Support Association survey of its members, most non-profit organizations consider their relationship with their local CCAC to be poor. Just over ten percent of them were willing to characterize the relationship as excellent. Commonly cited problems included CCACs' failure to refer people to them for community-support services, such as meals-on-wheels and friendly visiting. Idiosyncrasies and lack of communication emerged as the most urgent issues. Not wanting to appear "biased," one CCAC refused to communicate with non-profit organizations competing for service contracts in the RFP process, even when the matters to be discussed were unrelated to the contract. One interviewee stated that her organization was not allowed to leave pamphlets with clients describing the wide range of non-CCAC, community services that they provide as an organization, such as friendly visiting or congregate dining. The CCAC view, as it was explained to the interviewee, was that if the organization were to leave community-service pamphlets with clients, it might obtain an unfair competitive advantage, because clients could request to be served by a non-profit. Although CCACs are charged with the responsibility of being the single point of access for all community services, in reality only a small percentage of CCACs accept this responsibility as a part of their mandate. CCACs claim they are not directly funded to take on this responsibility.

From the perspective of the representatives of the community associations that we spoke with, two issues in particular are at the root of the problems in the relationship between the CCACs and the non-profit agencies. First, the provincial government has not provided the proper leadership in order to ensure that there is continuity of service between the CCACs and the voluntary non-profit organizations which are also funded by the Ministry. Secondly, each of the CCACs is unique and quite independent of the others. While this affords the potential to be very responsive to local needs, it may also give rise to idiosyncrasies.

In most cases, the actions of individual CCACs are partially driven by local needs on the one hand, and by a lack of policy direction, on the other. This lack of direction has resulted in a situation of *street-level bureaucracy*, wherein policy-making is not flowing down from the provincial level, but is being tailor-made in each instance. (Lipsky, 1980) The recent implementation of the *Community Care Access Corporations Act, 2001* (Bill 130), in December 2001, establishes more government control of CCACs, as both board members and Executive Directors are now Order in Council appointments. Whether this amounts to more complicity, more standardization across the province, or less activism on the part of CCACs, is yet to be determined.

The Changing Role of Non-Profit Organizations

Programmatic retrenchment has affected non-profit organizations in the home-care sector in subtle and profound ways, causing them to change the services they provide and how they spend their time. They are providing fewer uniquely local programs and services, instead choosing to concentrate on services for which they receive government funding. Services funded by government are being atrophied, redefined and pared down. For example, agencies are facing decisions about where an elderly frail senior can go with subsidized transportation, despite the fact that the client pays for a portion of the ride. Many organizations have very reluctantly decided to provide rides only to medical appointments, cancelling transportation to social-care activities. Interviewees indicate that transportation is but one example.

In profound ways organizations are changing the way they inter-act both with their peer organizations and with the state. Imposing a contractual, fee-for-service logic on organizations, and moving pro-fessional and paraprofessional services more fully into the market means that non-profits have needed to develop split personalities, operating by market imperatives and non-profit charitable imperatives simulta-neously. Some organizations have simply been unable to compete. Although the Red Cross and VON have provided home-care services for nearly a century, these organizations have been challenged to the core—from their organizational structure to the services they pro-vide—since 1999 when the reservation for non-profit providers was removed. They have been forced to restructure and to re-think how to "do business." Other non-profit organizations—Saint-Elizabeth Health Care, for example, have been quite successful.

Managed competition for professional and para-professional serv-ices and the *Planning Funding and Accountability Manual* are the cur-rent policy tools used by the Ontario government to govern the allo-cation of public dollars for home-care services. They are in place to ensure that services are delivered effectively, efficiently and with ac-countability. Casting to the side discussion of whether or not these are the correct policy goals to have, evidence suggests that these goals are not being met with the current policy tools.

Accountability is enforced with reporting, and the requirements on this score are quite burdensome for community support organiza-tions, even though these organizations account for a small portion of the overall home-care pie. By contrast, providers of home-care service contracts report only to the CCACs, and data regarding the price, number, and cost-effectiveness of their services are hidden from the public. CCACs are responsible for delivering services in the aggre-gate, but there is no way for the public to tell how individual provider organizations are faring. A comparison of CCAC annual reports from across the province reveals little consistency in approach. In the com-petitive environment, accountability to the public has actually been reduced. And while organizations may be reporting more numbers to the Ministry, since they are forced to game the system, and because not all organizations report units of service in the same way, the data that is gathered is not reliable in the aggregate for comparative purposes.

Home care in Ontario represents a very clear picture of programmatic retrenchment. Quite simply, the latter has changed which organizations receive public funding, how they apply to get their funding, what services they get money for, and how and what they report to the province. Interviewees feel that the policy tools that are being used by the Ministry stifle their creativity without noticeable gains to public accountability and efficiency in the use of public resources.

Conclusion

There are several important reasons to study home care in Ontario through the history of the relationship between the non-profit sector and the state. First, it is clear that non-profit organizations have historically depended on the state for their growth and expansion. Second, they developed their role as partners with the state during the growth of the welfare state. It was during this period that they actually enjoyed the most autonomy to pursue locally based social-welfare goals. Third, recent state retrenchment is not primarily a function of overt fiscal restraint but one of less obvious changes brought about by the centralization of authority, the standardization of services and programs across the province, and the restriction in the quantity and nature of publicly funded services.

Before1945, the state played a limited role in funding and delivering health and social care, while non-profit organizations were more active in that capacity. From 1945 until the mid-1970s, the state expanded into most areas of health and social care. This period is also characterized by the expansion and proliferation of non-profit voluntary organizations. Organizations flourished as the state spent more on health and social care. It was during this period that non-profit organizations acted as partners with government to carry out the tasks of welfare that exceeded the state role. A third historical period is marked by beginnings of the unravelling of the post-war welfare state, roughly corresponding to the period from the mid-1970s until the early 1990s. This was a gradual process, initially spurred by government's response to declining economic growth, high inflation rates, and high government debt. It was during this period that Ontario's health-and-social-care-delivery infrastructure came under increasing scrutiny. The Conservative government of the 1970s began to offload service-delivery functions to the private sector (voluntary non-profit sector, private business and individuals and families) and local levels of government. This decision supported a shift in the institutional focus of government and the bureaucracy, away from policies that supported the expansion of the service-delivery capacity of the state towards state retrenchment.

State retrenchment is literally a process of retreat, a shrinking of the role of the state. In the most recent period, the fiscal commitment of the provincial state to funding home-care services has masked the less obvious effects of programmatic retrenchment, which is not primarily a function of overt fiscal restraint, but of less obvious changes brought about by the restriction in the quantity and nature of publicly funded services. While the state is paying more, *what* is paid for has narrowed. And, by virtue of the downloading from hospitals to the community, health-care needs and services have trumped social care. The capacity of the state to act autonomously in this sector is great, due to the large degree of centralization of authority in the Ministry of Health and Long Term Care. Furthermore the ways in which the state ensures contract compliance and accountability have become more onerous for small grassroots organizations, while the data collected are no more revealing. As contractors of the state and competitors for state contracts, non-profit organizations continue to play a large role in social welfare, but their autonomy from the state has diminished. In the face of the human-resources crisis, the accountability requirements and the "street-level bureaucratic" policies adopted by individual CCACs, many non-profit organizations are feeling overwhelmed.

Programmatic retrenchment is affecting the nature and number of non-profit organizations and the community support services they provide. They have reported increased demands for their services. More time must be spent raising money from alternative sources, while fundraising needs are becoming more sophisticated as the field of competition grows.

The emergence of the competitive, managerial state, wedded to a competitive contract culture, has also facilitated a massive re-allocation of state resources from non-profit voluntary organizations to for-profit organizations. For professional and paraprofessional non-profits, the problem with the managed competition model is not so much that some organizations will not fare well. The major problem is that it forces organizations to be Janus-faced. They must accomplish the non-profit, community-focused goals they have set themselves, while achieving the objectives of providing a stipulated number of negotiated services established in their contracts with the CCAC or directly with the Ministry. While responding to opportunities to pursue their organizational missions through home-care service contracts with CCACs, they must be competitive and market-focused. At the same time, their mandates may require them to "pick-up" residual health and social care in their communities that cannot be provided by the institutional health-care system, by individuals or by their families. While they try to fill both the opportunities and gaps, they cannot let one side of their organization seep into the other. The benefit of being Janus-faced is that it affords perspective in both directions. The problem is that it may require choice, such that an organization can only take the middle path, or must split in order to do more than one thing well.

The shift in the role of the state—to contractor, regulator and partner—is resulting in several unwanted consequences for non-profit organizations, particularly if—as in the case of home care—the state does not support their autonomy, even as it needs to rely on them to deliver needed health and social care. Brooks warns that:

> [i]f governments continue to cut back on social services and to shift them to the voluntary sector, not only will they jeopardize the provision of these services and the social goals that they serve, but also they will produce a voluntary sector that will be largely passive and irrelevant, instead of being vital and innovative. Furthermore the apparently increasing prevalent view that "downsizing" government and increasing the

presence of voluntary organizations can revitalize civil society is profoundly wrong. An active and vibrant democratic government is a prerequisite for a flourishing civil society. (Brooks, 1999, p.166)

The case of home-care delivery in Ontario illustrates the transformation of the voluntary non-profit organizations' collective role *vis à vis* the state.

Variously described as *partners* or *gap fillers*, with their role described as *central, vital* or supporting *an emerging middle way*, voluntary non-profit organizations that provide health and social care have been left to respond to state retreat and retrenchment. They are burdened by the fact that they have moved from a role of partner with the state—identifying and filling the needs of local and particular populations—to being "just another private contractor" obliged to deliver specified services at a specified price, or to responding when none other is able. Ultimately, the massive program and system-level restructuring of the home-care sector in Ontario will have long-term implications for the overall character of the non-profit organizations that survive the shift in their relationship with the state.

Bibliography

Advisory Board on the Voluntary Sector (1997). *Report of the Advisory Board on the Voluntary Sector.* http://www.gov.on.ca/MBS/english/press/action.html (accessed on February 13th, 2001).

Baranek, P. M. (2000). *Long Term Care Reform in Ontario: The Influence of Ideas, Institutions and Interests on the Public/Private Mix*, Ph.D. thesis, Toronto, University of Toronto, Graduate Department of Health Administration.

Baranek, P. M., R. B. Deber, et al. (1999). "Policy Trade-offs in 'Home Care': the Ontario Example," *Canadian Public Administration*, 42:1, 69-92.

Bellamy, D. (1983). "Social Policy in Ontario," in *The Province of Ontario: Its Social Services*, Toronto, Ontario Social Development Council.

Brooks, Neil (1999). "The Role of the Voluntary Sector in a Modern Welfare State," in J. Phillips, B. Chapman & D. Stevens (eds.), *Between State and Mar-*

ket: Essays on Charities Law and Policy in Canada, Montreal, McGill-Queen's University Press, 166-218.

Browne, Paul Leduc (2000). *Unsafe Practices: Restructuring and Privatization in Ontario Health Care*, Ottawa, CCPA Books.

Browne, Paul Leduc (1996). *Love in a Cold World? The Voluntary Sector in an Age of Cuts*, Ottawa, Canadian Centre for Policy Alternatives.

Committee on Government Productivity (1971). *Interim Report No. 3*. Government of Ontario, 51.

Community Care Access Centre of Waterloo Region (2002). *Expenditure Control Plan Update*, Report to the Board of Directors, Waterloo, Community Care Access Centre of Waterloo Region.

Community Care Access Centre of Waterloo Region (2001a). *Expenditure Control Plan Update*, Report to the Board of Directors, Waterloo, Community Care Access Centre of Waterloo Region.

Community Care Access Centre of Waterloo Region (2001b). *Provincial Impacts of MOHLTC Funding Levels for Fiscal 2001: No Growth—Hold the Line on Service Levels*, Report to the Board of Directors, Waterloo, Community Care Access Centre of Waterloo Region.

Coyte, P. C., R. Hall & R. Croxford (1999). *Inter-Provincial Variation in Home Care Funding*, Toronto, Home Care Evaluation and Research Centre.

Daly, Tamara (2003). *The Grassroots Ceiling: The Impact of State Policy Change on Home Support Non-Profits in Ontario and in Waterloo Region - Wellington-Dufferin (1958 - 2001)*, Ph.D. thesis, Toronto, University Of Toronto, Department of Health Policy, Management and Evaluation, Faculty of Medicine, 342.

Daly, Tamara (2002). "Unearthing Grassroots? Voluntary Non-Profit Organizations in Ontario's Home Health and Social Care Sector," Paper presented at the Annual Meeting of the Canadian Political Science Association, Toronto, University of Toronto, May 30.

Deber, R. B. & A. P. Williams (1995). "Policy, Payment and Participation: Long-Term Care Reform in Ontario," *Canadian Journal on Aging*, 14:2, 294-318.

Dexter, B. (2001). "Is Nobody Home to Staff Home Care?" *Toronto Star*, May 5.

Drache, Daniel, Duncan Cameron & the Social Planning Council of Metro Toronto (1985), "The Rise and Fall of the Welfare State," in Duncan Cameron (ed.), *The Other Macdonald Report*, Toronto, James Lorimer & Company.

Dreessen, E. (2001). "What We Should Know About the Voluntary Sector But Don't," *ISUMA: Canadian Journal of Policy Research*, 2:2.

Drover, Glenn (1983). "Beyond the Welfare State: Brief to the Royal Commission on the Economic Union and Development Prospects for Canada," *The Social Worker*, 51:1.

Esping-Andersen, Gøsta (1990). *The Three Worlds of Welfare Capitalism*, Princeton, Princeton University Press.

Febbraro, A. R., M. Hall, et al. (1999). *Developing a Typology of the Voluntary Health Sector in Canada: Definition and Classification Issues*, Ottawa, Health Canada, Voluntary Health Sector Project. http://www.hc-sc.gc.ca/hppb/voluntarysector/pdf/5_1_h.pdf (accessed on April 14th 2001).

Flora, P. & J. Alber (1981). "Modernization, Democratization and the Development of Welfare States in Europe," in P. Flora and A. Heidenheimer (eds.), *The Development of Welfare States in Europe and America*, London, Transaction Books.

Guest, Dennis (1986). *The Emergence of Social Security in Canada*, Vancouver, UBC Press.

Hadley, Roger & Hatch, Stephen (1981). *Social Welfare and the Failure of the State*, London, Allen and Unwin.

Hall, Michael & Keith Banting (2000). "The Nonprofit Sector in Canada: An Introduction," in Keith Banting (ed.), *The Nonprofit Sector in Canada: Roles and Relationships*, Kingston, Queen's University School of Policy Studies.

Hall, Michael & Paul Reed (1998). "Shifting the Burden: How Much Can Government Download to the Non-Profit Sector?" *Canadian Public Administration*, 41:1.

Ham, C. (1997). "Lessons and Conclusions," in *Health Care Reform: Learning From International Experience*, Buckingham, Open University Press.

Health Canada (1990). *Report on Home Care*, prepared by the Federal/Provincial/Territorial Working Group on Home Care.

Hirdes, J., D. Dalby & J. Poss (2001). *The Use of Homemaking and Personal Support Services in the CCAC of Waterloo Region*, RAI Health Informatics Project (RAI-HIP), Waterloo, Department of Health Studies & Gerontology, University of Waterloo.

Hollander, Michael J. (1999). *Comparative Cost Analysis of Home Care and Residential Care Services - Preliminary Findings*, Health Transition Fund, Health Canada. http://www.homecarestudy.com (accessed on May 15th, 2001).

Hollander, Michael, Raisa Deber, et al. (2000). *Application of the Five Principles of the Canada Health Act to Home Care: Possibilities and Implications*, paper commissioned by the Canadian Nurses Association, January.

Interview 010902.

Interview 011402.

Interview 040202.

Interview 041702B.

Interview 051402.

Interview 051402B.

Interview 051502.

Interview 051602.

Jenson, Jane (1989). "'Different' but not 'Exceptional': Canada's Permeable Fordism," *Canadian Review of Sociology and Anthropology*, 26:1.

Jenson, Jane & Susan Phillips (2000). "Distinctive Trajectories: Home Care and the Voluntary Sector in Quebec and Ontario," in Keith Banting (ed.), *The Nonprofit Sector in Canada*, Kingston, Queen's University School of Policy Studies, 28-67.

Kelly, A. (2002). "VON loses contract, 60 jobs," *The Kitchener-Waterloo Record*, February 6, B1.

Lang, V. (1974). *The Service State Emerges in Ontario 1945-1973*, Toronto, Ontario Economic Council.

Lipsky, Michael (1980). *Street-Level Bureaucracy*, New York, Russell-Sage Foundation.

Marosi, N. (2001). "Preface," *Talking Health Care: Is Community Care At a Turning Point?* (transcript of the proceedings of a community forum), Waterloo, Community Care Access Centre of Waterloo Region.

Mishra, R., G. Laws & P. Harding (1988). "Ontario," in J. S. Ismael and Y. Vaillancourt (eds.), *Privatization and Provincial Social Services in Canada*, Edmonton, University of Alberta Press, 119 -139.

Moscovitch, Allan & Glenn Drover (1987). "Social Expenditure and the Welfare State: The Canadian Experience in Historical Perspective," in Allan Moscovitch & Jim Albert (eds.), *The Benevolent State: The Growth of Welfare in Canada*, Toronto, Garamond Press.

OACCAC (2001). *RFP Survey of CCACs*, Scarborough, Ontario Association of Community Care Access Centres .

OACCAC (2000). *Human Resources: A Looming Crisis in the Community Care System*, Ontario Association For Community Care Access Centres, July 26. http://www.oaccac.on.ca/papers/HR_Position_Paper.pdf (accessed May 14th, 2001).

OHHCPA (2001). *Private Sector Delivery of Home Health Care in Ontario*, Ontario Home Health Care Providers' Association, June. www.ohhcap.on.ca/ docs (accessed May 18th, 2001).

OECD (1997). *Societal Cohesion and the Globalizing Economy: What Does the Future Hold?* Paris, Organization for Economic Co-operation and Development.

Ontario (2001). *Community Care Connects!* Toronto, Ministry of Health and Long Term Care and CCACs. http://www.communitycareconnects.com/ home.asp, accessed on Sept 15th, 2001.

Ontario (1975). *The Report of the Special Program Review Committee*, Toronto, Government of Ontario.

The Peel Web, *The Old Poor Law 1795-1834,* http://www.adw03.dial.pipex.com/ peel/plaa.htm accessed on April 18, 2001.

Pierson, Paul (1994). *Dismantling the Welfare State? Reagan, Thatcher, and the Politics of Retrenchment*, New York, Press Syndicate of the University of Cambridge.

Price Waterhouse Coopers (2000). *A Review of Community Care Access Centres in Ontario: Final Report*, Toronto.

Price Waterhouse (1989). *Operational Review of the Ontario Home Care Program: Final Report*, Toronto, Price Waterhouse.

Putnam, Robert. D. (1993). *Making Democracy Work: Civic Traditions in Modern Italy*, Princeton, Princeton University Press.
Rekart, Josephine (1993). *Public Funds, Private Provision. The Role of the Voluntary Sector*, Vancouver, UBC Press.

Rice, James J. & Michael J. Prince (2000). *Changing Politics of Canadian Social Policy*, Toronto, University of Toronto Press.

Salamon, Lester (1995). *Partners in Public Service*, Baltimore, The Johns Hopkins University Press.

Soo, K. (2001). "Red Cross Workers in Limbo," *Toronto Star*, B2.

Stein, Janice G. (2001). *The Cult of Efficiency*, Etobicoke, Anansi.

Taylor, Malcolm (1987). *Health Insurance and Canadian Public Policy*, Kingston, McGill-Queen's University Press.

The Johns Hopkins Comparative Nonprofit Sector Project. http://www.jhu.edu/~cnp/research.html(accessed on March 26th, 2001).

Tindale, J. & E. MacLachlan (2001). "VON 'doing commercial': The Experience of Executive Directors with Related Business Development," in Kathy Brock & Keith Banting (eds.), *The Nonprofit Sector and Government in a New Century*, Kingston, McGill-Queen's University Press.

Toronto District Health Council and Toronto Area Community Care Access Centres (2000). *Service Utilization Patterns in Community Care Access Centres in Toronto 1996 - 1999.*

Tuohy, Carolyn (1999). *Accidental Logics: The Dynamics of Change in the Health Care Arena in the United States, Britain, and Canada*, New York, Oxford University Press.

United Way of Greater Toronto (1997). *Metro Toronto: A Community at Risk*, Toronto, United Way of Greater Toronto.

VHA Home Health Care (2001). *Service Trends for CCAC Clients 1998, 1999, 2000 and PSW Compensation Comparison.* http://www.vha.ca/news/servicetrend.htm (accessed on April 30th, 2001).

VON Canada (2003). "VON Waterloo-Wellington-Dufferin Branch to Close," www.von.ca/english/News/WWD2003.htm.

Wellington-Dufferin CCAC (2002). "Nursing Services Contracts Awarded," Community Care Access Centre of Wellington-Dufferin.

Waterloo & Wellington - Dufferin District Health Councils (1997/1998). *Waterloo Region and Wellington and Dufferin Counties CCAC Service Utilization Profile.*

Williams, A. M. (1996). "The Development of Ontario's Home Care Program: A Critical Geographical Analysis," *Social Science and Medicine*, 42:6, 937-948.

Williams, A. P., J. Barnsley, S. Leggat, R. B. Deber & P. Baranek (1999). "Long Term Care Goes to Market: Managed Competition and Ontario's Reform of Community Based Services," *Canadian Journal on Aging*, 18:2, 125-51.

Williams, A.P., R. Deber, et al. (2001). "From Medicare to Home Care: Globalization, State Retrenchment and the Profitization of Canada's Health Care System," in Pat Armstrong, Hugh Armstrong & David Coburn (eds.), *Unhealthy Times: Political Economy Perspectives on Health Care in Canada*, Don Mills, Oxford University Press, 7-30.

Wolch (1990). *The Shadow State: Government and Voluntary Sector in Transition*, New York, The Foundation Centre.

Notes

[1] This paper expands and refines a paper I initially presented at the Canadian Sociology and Anthropology Association meeting in Quebec with Professors A.P. Williams and Raisa Deber. (Daly, 2001) It stems from my doctoral research. I would like to acknowledge the financial support of a Doctoral Fellowship from the National Health Research and Development Program/Canadian Institutes for Health Research, and an M-THAC Opportunities Grant for the transcription of the interviews. Thank you to all of the inter-

viewees, who have been generous with their time, their knowledge and their support of the research. I am also very thankful to Dr. Raisa Deber, my supervisor, for her thoughtful comments and suggestions. I would also like to thank Dr. Paul Leduc Browne and the anonymous reviewers for their constructive editorial comments. Thank you to Dr. A. P. Williams and Dr. J. Lum for their comments on an early draft. I wish to acknowledge and thank my family and close friends for their support, and notably my parents and grandparents, who took the time to read this chapter and make comments, and who have always shown an enduring interest in my academic pursuits. Thank you to Dr. J.D. Maggi for her constructive feedback and valuable insight. My deepest gratitude is reserved for my husband Chris Ullock as it is his love, intellectual support and feedback that I rely upon the most. All failings remain my responsibility.

2   Pierson sees systematic retrenchment taking place outside of the boundary of the welfare state, but Rice and Prince argue that in Canada the welfare state is embedded within society and the economy. Rice and Prince (2000) also see *paradigmatic retrenchment* as a third category in which support for the guiding principle of state intervention in the economy and society is dropped or reduced.

3   This chapter draws on the content analysis of forty-eight interviews with key informants in several large, urban, multi-service organizations, with current and former members of the Ministry of Health and Long Term Care, and with District Health Council representatives and with sector associations. I have relied on supporting documentary evidence and figures from the Community Support Services Administrative Database, and on secondary published data. Unfortunately, longitudinal data on individual organizations within this sector are unavailable. (Dreessen, 2001) Despite the need for good home-care sector data, it is difficult to obtain, for a variety of reasons. Data collected and stored by the Ministry is questionable after 1995, since the data in the Ontario Home Care Administrative System (OHCAS), the provincial data warehouse for the home-care system, is not considered very reliable (Interview, 080801). As well, information collected by private companies with public CCACs home-care contracts is proprietary. There is reportedly wide variation in the contracting process used by the different CCACs, making easy comparisons between different CCACs difficult. (PriceWaterhouseCoopers, 2000) This finding is also borne out in a review of CCACs' annual reports from 1996/1997 to 2000/2001. There is a great deal of variability in the manner in which CCACs report and disclose information to their communities, even on very simple items such as the age categories of those admitted to the CCAC. Comparative statistics about each of the CCACs are not easily obtained. Nor are common measurements or definitions used to track and assess management or clinical performance. As well, there are differences in the level of coopera-

tion between the CCACs and their District Health Councils. In some cases, the latter have cooperated with the CCACs to produce excellent reports about home-care service utilization. (Waterloo & Wellington-Dufferin District Health Councils, 1997-98; Toronto District Health Council, 2000) However, this is not the case across the province. The result of lack of directions at the provincial level and the paucity of good data on which to base decisions is that it is very difficult to get a handle on what has happened in this sector since the introduction of managed competition. While many of the data problems may be ironed out if the *Community Care Connects!* information system project is fully implemented, the reality is that data from the period 1995/1996 until the present is not entirely reliable. (Ontario, 2001)

[4] The Poor Law established local religious parishes as the unit of governance for the purposes of relief of poverty, and relied on the judgment of unpaid, non-professional administrators. Since local parishes were small and their sources of finance were unsteady, unusually heavy burdens such as those experienced between 1815 and 1821 proved disastrous for some parishes. Although there was not a single consistent body of practical application of the Poor Laws in England between 1601 and 1834, they had a profound overarching institutional effect on other laws. For instance, they had the effect of rationalizing some local practices, including the implementation of the 1662 Settlement Laws that required the practice of returning poor paupers to the parish of their birth. The law required residence of a year and a day for a person to qualify for relief. Subsequent amendments to the laws were also variations on the notion that the poor belonged to the place of their birth, or that they were not eligible for relief until a sufficient amount of time had passed. (The Peel Web, 2001)

[5] They indicate that the following problems might occur: the agency could provide more nursing visits than may be required; nurses might be employed to provide service where a less qualified and less expensive resource would suffice; there could be a tendency towards longer lengths of stay in the program; and finally, the HCPs' eligibility criteria might be applied less stringently, given the philosophy of right to treatment espoused by the VON.

[6] Federal commitment to health-care funding had already been reduced in 1977 when the federal government moved from a 50/50 cost-sharing formula for health care and post-secondary to a block grant under *Established Programs Financing* (EPF).

[7] Under the terms of the *Canada Health Act, 1984* (CHA), there are two categories of health-care services: "insured services" and "extended health-care services." Insured services are hospital services, physician services and surgical dental services that are provided in a hospital setting. Extended health-care services include nursing-home intermediate care services, adult residential-care services, home-care services and ambulatory health-care serv-

ices. In order to retain eligibility for federal Canada Health and Social Transfer funding, provinces and territories are required to comply with the five principles of the Canada Health Act (public administration, comprehensiveness, universality, portability and accessibility) for insured services. Provinces/territories are exempt from complying with the five principles for extended health-care services, although provinces may choose to fund these extended services depending on their own spending priorities and prerogatives. Under the rubric of publicly funded "extended health-care services," home-care services are not subject to the five principles of Medicare. Since home care is exempt from complying with the five principles, each province/territory retains decision-making authority to determine whether or not to fund home-care services. In reality, all provinces fund some home-care services, although the extent of funding has resulted in a great deal of variation between provinces/territories.

[8] Voluntary non-profit organizations may receive MOHLTC funding indirectly, in the form of service contracts with CCACs and/or directly from the Ministry for community support services based on service agreements. Residual health and social services are met with a combination of federal funding, private donations, United Way grants, and user fees. Remaining needs of clients in the community are either met through informal networks of families and friends, clients' return to hospital, placement in long-term-care facilities, or are not at all.

[9] The percentage of nursing *hours* done by non-profits has declined by 20 percentage points, but their share of RPN *hours* has actually grown by 7 percentage points. (Figure 3) Although RPN home *visits* increased in absolute terms by nearly 11 percent between 1995 and 2000, the number of *hours* they spent in the home skyrocketed by 188 percent. The opposite is true of RNs. The total number of RN visits increased by 29 percent, but the total number of hours they spent on them did not keep pace, increasing by only 14 percent.

Chapter 3
The Welfare State in Retreat: The Impact of Home-Care Restructuring on Women's Labour[1]
Allison Williams

Introduction

For decades the public sector has provided full-time and relatively well-paid jobs for women, who have also benefitted from the pay equity programs that are more likely to apply to public than private employment. Not only has the expanded public sector provided women with an important source of employment, but through the union movement, it has also been an important site for improvements in wage and working conditions. In addition, public-sector programs have helped to alleviate the many contradictory demands on women, by relieving some of the burdens of the double day. Women not only deliver welfare services, but are also their chief consumers, although often on behalf of others, such as ageing parents.

At the same time, the services and policies of the welfare state frequently incorporate significant, though implicit, assumptions about gender roles and thus actively shape gender relations. The ease or difficulty with which women can enter paid work, the way in which the unpaid work of caring for others is treated, and the regulation of marital and family relationships, are all central arenas where gender relations are constituted, and these are all influenced in significant ways by the nature and extent of state intervention. (Orloff, 1993) Social structures, values and attitudes persistently produce occupational segregation—the tendency for women to have different roles than men. Space and place (i.e. local context) are also clearly implicated in the social construction of occupational segregation. (Hanson and Pratt, 1995; Massey, 1995; Sheppard and Barnes, 1990; Thrift and Williams, 1987; Walker, 1985)

Occupational segregation begins at home, as women's labour-market positions are linked to their household responsibilities. Paid caregiving appears as an outgrowth of women's traditional role; it is the result of sex-role stereotyping which places women in jobs that are extensions of their personal lives (Pines et al., 1981): "... care giving transcends the bifurcation between public and private. Women perform similar care-giving activities in the domestic domain and the public arena." (Abel and Nelson, 1990, 6) Home care accentuates the merging of public and private, as care is given solely in the home. This is especially true for the paid work of home-support workers, as normally unpaid domestic tasks are performed in the home. Like all caregiving work done in capitalist society, formal care in the home is subordinated and devalued in the marketplace when it is done for a wage. Among the various explanations of the ways in which women participate as a segregated group in the labour force (Kobayashi, 1994), the traditional division of labour best fits the work situation of home-care practitioners.

Cuts in state support for social and health programs over the past decade have resulted in the implementation of various restructuring strategies, which have had a negative impact on women's paid and unpaid work. (Peck, 1996; McDowell, 1994, 1989;Webster, 1985) Women comprise the bulk of the producers of the public services that have been cut (Webster, 1985) and dominate many of the occupations indirectly funded by the welfare state, such as health care. The restructuring taking place in women's work in the home and in the workplace has intensified the experience of the double day. (Luxton and Reiter, 1997; Brodie, 1994) Women bear a disproportionate share of the costs of restructuring; and class and race interrelate with gender to further disadvantage women.

Not-for-profit home-care agencies are particularly relevant in this context, because they have traditionally been funded mainly by public monies and have, in many cases, operated very much like a public service. Not-for-profit agencies have traditionally provided higher rates of pay and better benefits than have the for-profit home-care agencies, and have had a proven reputation for maintaining service standards and quality care. Restructuring has affected the "good" jobs more dramatically than those traditionally understood to have low occupational status. These changes have exacerbated shortages in medically under-serviced areas and have had significant effects on the labour process, as well as on the time-space relations of practitioners' work.

The adoption of new labour processes is often driven by financial factors, although types of management, labour relations, and the size of organizations may also play a role. (Massey, 1995) Under capitalism, the special nature of labour power as a commodity makes the labour process a focal point for analyzing reform. Labour process analysis brings to light the nature, mechanisms and processes of power and control in paid work. The transformation of the labour process is apparent in shifting work structures, functions, conditions, and expectations—all of which affect the quality of working life for formal practitioners, not to mention the quality of care provided to clients. Working conditions include job demands, role characteristics, organizational characteristics and policies, and the physical surroundings in which an individual works, which could be unduly hazardous or detrimental to health (because of excessive noise, air pollution, heat or cold, for example). (Brief et al., 1981)

In the 1990s, like the majority of Western countries, Canada moved away from institutional care towards a home-based care system in order to save money. (Lesemann and Martin, 1993) In the last two decades, most Western countries initiated spending constraints on institutional care. France, the Netherlands, and Sweden, for example, all did this in the early 1980s. (Monk and Cox, 1991) This coincided with the promotion, and increasing availability, of a growing variety of home-care services. The Western World has experienced a broad shift in the geography of care, from centralized, hospital-based care to decentralized, home-based care. To further limit spending, "cost-efficient" strategies have also been implemented within home-care systems:

> ... reducing certain benefits, limited access to certain services and decentralizing their management, privatization approaches, allocation of financial aid to individuals to enable them to purchase what they need in the service market, etc. There is also broader use of evaluation procedures to enhance

and monitor professional and organizational efficiency, by comparing their objectives, methods and performance. Finally, we might point to attempts to highlight the contribution already being offered or that could potentially be supplied by front-line resources: families, friends and neighbourhoods, as well as peer self-help at the home or community level, which provide a form of primary care. (Lesemann and Martin, 1993, vii)

In Ontario, the cuts of the 1990s, together with deficit-cutting provincial reforms involving de-institutionalization and hospital restructuring, had a negative impact on home care—the fastest growing long-term-care service in the province. (White, 1994) At the same time that greater demands for increasingly complex care were being felt in the home-care sector, costs were being cut in a variety of ways. Because of a failure of funding to keep up with the demand for services, care had to be rationed. This clearly had an impact on its quality. Furthermore, increased demands and diminishing resources took their toll on formal caregivers, particularly nurses.

Care for the elderly and other dependent populations clearly illustrates the impact of the retreat of the welfare state on women's paid and unpaid work. The transfer of elderly caregiving responsibilities to informal (unpaid) caregivers reveals state assumptions about women's availability and obligation to care. Cuts in public provision shift the work of eldercare to families, demonstrating how capitalism reorganizes the labour process to make use of free labour. (Glazer, 1993) Community-based services are increasingly only provided to buttress and sustain family carers, not to substitute for them. The vast majority of eldercare is carried out by women, as women do more tasks, spend more time, have a greater sense of obligation, and experience more stress in caring for elderly kin than do men. (Medjuck et al., 1992)

Although not-for-profit home-care agencies for the most part had excellent employment practices, they were compelled to adopt new management programs. They experienced:

- closer scrutiny of the delivery of cost-saving and appropriate services;
- increasing competition from other service agencies, which demanded clear evidence of quality;
- ongoing pressures for fiscal accountability and tighter financial management; and
- changing demand patterns as knowledgeable customers analyzed and challenged the health-care system. (Green et al., 1994)

As the wages of practitioners make up the bulk of the agencies' costs, the latter "[were] shifted to paid home-care providers who [were], for the most part, cheaper, less well-organized, and more isolated than their institutional counterparts and, thus, more open to exploitation." (Aronson and Neysmith, 1997, 47) Although the intended impact of restructuring was clearly met, as money was saved and the deficit reduced at both the federal and provincial levels, the transformation of the labour process fundamentally reshaped home-care practitioners' lives. (Connelly, 1995)

Because welfare arrangements and restructuring strategies vary so much across space, a geographical perspective is essential to their understanding. (Pinch, 1997) In the mid-1990s, I carried out a study of the impact of restructuring on home-care workers in Northern Ontario, a highly rural region consisting of 86 percent of the province's total land area but only 10 percent of its population—much of which resides in the small towns that dominate the landscape.[2] (Beggs, 1991) This region had been labelled "medically under-serviced," as it had traditionally experienced a shortage of specialty services and human-health-care resources. Restructuring further affected the female-dominated health-care sector, and home care in particular. The history of home care in Ontario makes clear that this northern region continues to be under-serviced, as all provincial home-care programs evolved in the south and were thereby shaped for and by a well serviced, densely populated region; the specific cultural and geographic needs of the northern region have still to be addressed. (Williams, 1996)

Occupational Segmentation in Home Care

There was a division of labour within the home-care workforce I studied (Figure 1). Registered nurses (RNs) were higher on the medical health hierarchy and had higher status than registered practical nurses (RPNs), while the latter enjoyed higher status than home-support workers (HSWs). The differences between the practitioner groups were reflected in each group's educational status, pay and authority.

RNs either had a university degree (3-4 years) or a college certificate acquired from two to three years of education, whereas RPNs had a college certificate after one year of education. The salaries and benefits of RNs and RPNs working in home care were lower than those of their hospital counterparts. (Konka, 1995) The majority of RNs and RPNs in the home-care sector were unionized and had professional associations. Although RNs and RPNs had traditionally had full-time employment, many were now part of a flexible work force

---

Figure 1: The Home Care Occupational Hierarchy

Physicians

Provincial Home Care Program
(Management, Case Assessment Officers, Health Specialists)

Agency Management

Supervisors

Other Specialists

Agency Management

Case Managers

Registered Nurses

Registered Practical Nurses

Home support workers

due to an increase in the proportion of permanent part-time workers, or made up a casual labour pool. (Armstrong and Armstrong, 1990) Because these two groups had a lot in common when compared with HSWs, they were pooled together in the survey analysis to avoid the problem of small sample sizes.

HSWs were paid much lower wages than nurses and often had limited benefits. (Oriol, 1985) Home-support workers had no professional association, most were non-unionized, and they were frequently hired as permanent part-time employees, "constituting a flexible pool of labour, a floating reserve." (Armstrong and Armstrong, 1990, 86) Like the other two groups of home-care practitioners, HSWs often had demanding schedules, rarely having two days off in a row and often working on weekends.

Among these workers, there was a direct relationship between occupational and socio-economic status. (Brown and Scase, 1991) As Rose (1993) and Massey (1995) both pointed out, diversity among women exists in the experience of paid work and of unpaid reproductive work, "most particularly along the lines of sexuality and ethnicity, as well as of class." (Massey, 1995, 354) Occupational segmentation in health care is structured by gender and "race":

> Those at the bottom of the pay scale, clerical and service "support" workers, are women and minority men, and conventionally regarded as peripheral to actual care giving. Those at the top are white and mainly male medical and managerial staff, who together with underpaid predominantly white women registered nurses (RNs) are seen as central to care delivery. The resulting pay and status hierarchy is both rigid and visible, with women and minority men almost absent from its well-paid upper levels, and white men few and far between at the bottom. (Sacks, 1990, 188)

The subordinate position of home-health-care practitioners reflects the occupational segmentation that is also found within the home-health-care environment. RNs, RPNs and HSWs have comparatively little prestige and status (Fisher, 1990; Butter et al., 1985), as they are all female and located at the bottom of the human home-health-care hierarchy.

A number of HSWs in my study were French Canadian, Aboriginal or represented various other national and ethnic identities. Only the Italian ethnic group was more strongly represented by nurses due to the long history of Italian-Canadian settlement throughout northern Ontario. (Algoma District Health Council, 1996) (Table 1) The greater representation of HSWs in ethnic groups other than English Canadian further indicates that class and race interrelate with gender to further disadvantage women. The lower occupational status characteristic of the HSW group is consistent with the experience of ethnic minorities (Brown and Scase, 1991; Littler and Salaman, 1984) and immigrant women. (Donovan, 1989)

Age is also a factor in the labour forces of different service industries. Younger working-class women are found in more glamorous

TABLE 1:Demographic Characteristics of Questionnaire Survey Respondents

CHARACTERISTIC	PRACTITIONER GROUP	
	NURSES [%] (n=131)	HOME SUPPORT WORKERS [%] (n=353)
EDUCATION		
grade 8 or less	-	8
high school	-	49
community college	68	0
university	23	9
graduate school	5	0
INCOME		
less than $10,000	0	5
$10-29,999	10	36
$30-49,999	23	35
$50-69,999	32	18
$70-79,999	35	6
MAJOR WAGE EARNER IN FAMILY	31	27
ETHNICITY		
English Canadians	65	55
AGE		
median	39	44
MARITAL AND FAMILY STATUS		
widowed	2	6
married	75	68
have children	80	87
children still at home (of those who have children)	91	68

NOTE:Characteristics in italics are significantly different (p < 0.05) between practitioner groups according to Mann-Whitney U tests.

service work, while older working-class women's choices revolve primarily around commodified forms of domestic work, including: "privatized cleaning services; kitchen domestic work and care work in relation to the elderly and mentally and/or physically disabled." (Gregson and Lowe, 1994, 128) HSWs in our sample were significantly older than the nurses. The fact that the HSWs were an older group is reflected in their marital status, as 6 percent of the sample was widowed. Fewer HSWs than nurses were married, although the majority of practitioners in both groups were living the double day—coming home from work to care for children. The number of children each practitioner group had remaining at home reflected the age differences between groups, as younger nurses were still in their childbearing years, while children of the relatively older HSWs had left or were leaving home.

Working Conditions

Job stress is an important element in job satisfaction—defined as an attitude people have toward their work. Stress occurs when people see environmental conditions as threats to their continued well-being. (Hudson & Sullivan, 1990) Job stress varies with status, as low-status occupations are associated with high levels of job stress. (Brief et al., 1981) RNs could therefore be expected to have the greatest job satisfaction—having the best working conditions and least amount of job stress—of the three practitioner groups, followed by RPNs, and finally, HSWs. (Esland and Salaman, 1980) However, restructuring challenged these well-known relationships among the workers surveyed.

Nurses' mean scores on the "working conditions" factor of our study were significantly ($p < 0.05$) less favourable than those of HSWs, indicating that nurses were less satisfied with their working conditions than HSWs.[3] This is evident in the significantly different ways in which they rated the five main criteria on which they were questioned (see Table 2 and 3): "chances for promotion are good", "respected by community members", "job security is good", "enjoy commuting between clients", and "hours are flexible and convenient".

Nurses suffered from a comparative lack of flexibility and convenience in work hours, because they worked in shifts and for longer hours (28 hours per week on average, versus 25 hours per week for HSWs). HSWs worked only in the daytime, while nurses were on days and nights. Forty percent of the nurses, but only 32 percent of the HSWs, worked between 30 and 39 hours per week. Only 4 percent of HSWs worked 40 or more hours per week, whereas 10 percent of the nurses did. The difference in hours between the two practitioner groups was also reflected in the number of additional hours that practitioners would have liked to work, as HSWs wished to work more additional hours than did the nurses.

The growing numbers of casual and part-time nurses were frustrated with their hours, as the qualitative data show. The agency adjusted their labour inputs over time to meet fluctuations in output. (Pinch, 1997) They were dissatisfied with the small number of hours they were receiving, the lack of control they felt they had over their work schedule, and the way their work interfered with their desired lifestyle:

> (...) the dissatisfaction (...) unstable work schedule due to my casual status. And I absolutely detest calling in at 11 am in the morning to say "do you have anything for this evening or for tomorrow," and not being able to go and have a day that I can go somewhere, because I have to stay around in case they call me. [RN3, FG2]

By contrast, the HSWs, all of whom were employed part-time, had more control over their work schedules. They were very grateful for the flexibility of their work hours, as it enabled them to meet their family responsibilities:

> They [management] let me choose my own hours. They're pretty flexible, like. If you want to work just mornings, you can work just mornings. If you want to work full-time, if the clients are there, she'll let you work full-time. Being able to get the days off when you want them, especially when you got smaller kids, like when Wayne was little, he got sick, and

I needed to know that I can take the time off and not lose my job... [HMKa, FG4]

It seems as though HSWs had more of a participatory role in determining their work hours than nurses did. Management would work around HSWs' requests, trying to ensure hours were rearranged, not reallocated. This did not seem to be the case for nurses, who are comparatively more expensive to employ, as the management appeared to have become more rigid about work schedules. This confirms that the relations between management and labour are implicated in the adoption of new labour processes, as Massey has suggested (1995).

Differences in the two groups' evaluations of their working conditions may also have had to do with the group(s) to which they compared themselves. (Romero, 1994) For example, home-care nurses may have assessed their working conditions with reference to those experienced by hospital nurses or their own managers. They may have viewed their working conditions as less satisfactory than those of comparable health-care professionals. By contrast, HSWs may have felt particularly satisfied about their work when comparing it to other employment opportunities that are open to them, as stated by one focus group participant:

It pays more than if you went for waitressing, or cleaning rooms, or whatever. It's above minimum wage, so if you don't have any skills and you can get into a job like this, then it's great, because you only have your home skills, eh? [HMKe, FG4]

Job Stress

My research showed that the nurses also experienced significantly more job stress ($p = .001$) than HSWs did. This is evident in the significantly different ways in which they rated the four main criteria on which they were questioned (see Table 3): "have enough time to get job done," "job responsibilities are decreasing," "work is not stressful," and "job requires resourcefulness." Although ratings of the fifth item, "are not supervised too closely," are not statistically significant, nurses also indicated less satisfaction on that score than HSWs did.

Nurses expressed a much higher level of disagreement than HSWs with the statement "job responsibilities are decreasing." Changes in the labour process increased nurses' responsibility for complex and technologically demanding job tasks. The transfer of patients from institutional to home care translated into a larger number of sophisticated skills in the home, as pointed out by a RN:

> (...) when I started 10 years ago with [name of agency], the type of call [was] totally different than what we are getting now. We [now] have all kinds of programs that were unheard of 10 years ago. We do a lot of high-tech work in the homes (...) we are now perfectly capable of doing it and are doing it. We're doing the IVs, we're doing the dialysis, those kinds of things; we do a lot more in the homes as opposed to educating. [RNd, FG2]

Such shifts in workload are becoming more frequent across the public sector, as Pinch (1997) has noted in his discussion of "functional flexibility," in which firms extend the range of their workers' skills and break down the barriers between different occupations.

Nurses did not always feel confident about their knowledge of complex skills. This was particularly the case for RNs who were assigned to overnight "on-call" duty:

> Well you know I find that there's some girls that know all these technical skills and they're doing them everyday and then there's all of us girls, the RNs that are on night call and have this same big fear of being called out to change a[n IV] pump (...) or something like that and not having a clue of what to do. And we all have to take our turn on night call (....) when I put that beeper on at 11 pm till 7-8 in the morning, I'm on call; anything can happen and there's tons of anxiety there, and yet I'm not alone. [RNc, FG1]

The lack of confidence felt by many nurses was blamed on lack of training: "(...) you are all supposed to handle any situation so they have you do a little quickie [training] session and say okay, you can do it, you're okay." [RNc, FG1] Dealing with increasing work responsibilities without proper training added to job stress.

As a result of cost pressures, job responsibilities increased while time allowances for patient visits decreased. The implementation of increasingly constraining time limits added to practitioners' job stress. The two practitioner groups differed significantly in their attitudes toward the time available to complete a job, as measured by the item "have enough time to get job done." Because they are more expensive to employ than HSWs, nurses had to cope with time constraints more than HSWs did. According to the nurses, cost-saving strategies translated into the intensification of work, defined as increases in labour productivity via managerial and organizational changes. (Massey, 1995) The enhanced intensification of work experienced by nurses has been identified as one of the most important changes affecting public-sector workers in recent years. (Pinch, 1997)

Time limitations, in addition to increasing job responsibilities of a sophisticated nature, contributed to practitioners' job stress, as measured by the item "work is not stressful." The significant difference in practitioners' assessments, with nurses feeling more job stress than HSWs, reflected the comparatively greater time-space constraints experienced by nurses. To quote one of the RNs in the study:

(...) they'll [home care agency] give you 6 patients that are all (...) needy in the afternoon and like they're supposed to spread out for the whole day, but you cannot fit 6 people in the morning and you know that the last one is going to be chomping at the bit when you walk in the door or you're even afraid to phone them because you don't want to tell them that you can't make it 'til 1 pm. So you just zip right through lunch and skip all your coffee breaks trying to get these 6 morning patients in 4 hours—now that's stress (....). [RNe, FG1]

Although home care practitioners may be able to do more than one task at once, they cannot be in more than one time or place at once.

Driving from one household to another complicates the time-space constraints that practitioners are experiencing as a result of work intensification and enhanced functional flexibility. Although management may wish for time-space convergence or the shrinking of distance in terms of the time needed to move between different locations (Janelle, 1969), the time it takes to drive from household A to household B has not changed as a result of reform (speed limits remain unchanged!). An RPN discussed her sense of dissatisfaction with time expectations given the spatial challenges she faces:

> What I'm not satisfied with (...) is the limited time we get; thirteen people in a day and you have half an hour for each person and that includes traveling time and, quite often I'm in about four or five different [geographical] areas in one day, and I could spend ten minutes with each person and still not make up my time (...) [RPNa, FG2]

An RN had a different response to the time-constraints:

> The time limit now—I don't even bother with the time limit; I do my thing and if I go over and I don't care about it and I just get paid for what they're going to pay me anyway; but I do feel good at the end of the day; I don't feel short-changed or anything. I'm not rushing anymore. [RNc, FG1]

As a result, this latter nurse would work a longer day, beyond the hours for which she is paid. This illustrates the way health-care costs get shifted to home-care practitioners as a result of labour-process change.

Increasing job stress and declining working conditions may have negative effects on employee retention, as job satisfaction, defined both in terms of working conditions and job stress, is related directly to turnover. Better working conditions would enhance workforce retention. (Canadian Nurses Association and Canadian Hospital Association, 1990) Job stress has been found to be an important reason why nurses leave the profession (Employment and Immigration Canada, 1989; Goldfarb Corporation, 1988), and may explain why nurses in the sample had been working fewer years than HSWs. This finding informs the acute shortage of nurses being experienced today in Ontario and across the country.

Although the difference in age across the two practitioner groups may have contributed to the variations evident in job tenure, with HSWs being significantly older than nurses and thereby being employed longer, job stress undoubtedly played a role. Forty percent of HSWs in the sample had been working for thirteen years or more, whereas only twenty-eight percent of the nurses had been employed that long. Sixty-eight percent of the nurses had been working for the same home-care agency for four years or less, whereas only fifty-seven percent of the HSWs had been employed by the same agency within the previous four years. Nurses were carrying out more complex tasks, working more intensively, and working longer hours than HSWs. The comparatively greater stress experienced by nurses may have been one of the factors contributing to their comparatively short job tenure. This was problematic in the medically under-serviced region of northern Ontario, which had difficulty recruiting and retaining health-care practitioners, such as nurses.

Conclusions

One of the surprising consequences of reform brought to light by my Northern Ontario study was the differential impact of restructuring on individual practitioner groups. Time-space constraints were implemented more intensively for nurses than for HSWs, because of nurses' higher wages. Nurses were forced to serve more patients in less time (intensification of work), while being given increased responsibility for tasks (functional flexibility). Despite being the occupational group with the highest status of the three studied, they experienced poorer working conditions, more job stress, and thereby worse job satisfaction than HSWs, the practitioner group with the relatively lower occupational status. This was unexpected, given the proven inverse relationship that generally prevails between occupational status on the one hand, and job stress, poor working conditions, and low job satisfaction on the other. A similar phenomenon has been observed among physicians in New Zealand (Kearns and Barnett, 1992) and other groups of health professionals throughout the western world. Perhaps the higher-status occupations are feeling the impacts of restructuring more, because they begin with higher expectations and thereby have further to fall. The HSWs are already at the bottom of the health-care hierarchy, being employed as part-time, non-unionized and poorly paid caregivers; consequently, their expectations are comparatively lower than their co-workers.

The restructuring process at work in the agencies I studied had a negative impact on the work lives of home-health-care practitioners, although it affected the various practitioner groups in different ways. My research suggests that changes to the welfare state in the 1990s turned back the clock on improving the lives of women. Women's paid home-care work became less stable and more intense, and, consequently, was characterized by increased job stress and poorer working conditions.

Appendix

This research employed both qualitative and quantitative methods, which included four focus groups, the results of which informed a mail-out questionnaire survey. The focus group discussions were made up of 6-10 practitioners from one of the two agencies (two groups were made up of RNs and RPNs and two groups were made up of HSWs). The semi-directed focus group discussions took place in the summer of 1993 and broadly defined work-life issues, which were then explored in greater detail in the questionnaire survey, which was implemented in the summer of 1994. All the respondents were women, as at the time of data collection, no men were employed in either of the home-care agencies concerned. All practitioners working in the two largest not-for-profit home-care agencies (one agency employing RNs and RPNs, and the other employing HSWs) were asked to participate in the questionnaire survey (n=1,157), which achieved a 42 percent response rate. No private, for-profit home-care agencies— which at the time had comparatively fewer practitioners than the non-profit agencies—were researched, as the focus of the research was on the agencies which provided publicly-funded services. Of the 484 respondents, 70 percent were HSWs, 8 percent RPNs and 15 percent RNs. To avoid the problems of small samples and to insure reliability, responses from RNs and RPNs were pooled together. Practitioners' assessments of work life were examined using a scale composed of 22 items. Each item is a work-related statement with which practitioners expressed their agreement using four standardized response categories: strongly agree (1), moderately agree (2), moderately disagree (3), and strongly disagree (4).

Using exploratory factor analysis with oblique rotation, the relationships among the 22 work-life items were interpreted by reducing the items into a few factors, defined as an underlying concept tapped into by the variables that are contained within it. (Alan & Duncan, 1990) The final rotated solution was restricted to three factors, each with an eigenvalue close to or greater than one. Factor 1 had the largest eigenvalue value (2.94), followed by Factor 2 (1.23) and finally, by Factor 3: (0.76). The three factors accounted for 24 percent of the variance, so their limited explanatory value has to be emphasized. Factors were interpreted based on items with substantial loadings (large absolute +/- values), which reflect the strength of the association between individual items and factors. (Alan and Duncan, 1990) Items with minor loadings were ignored in the interpretation of the factors. (Kim and Mueller, 1978) The three factors describing related items were identified as follows: Factor 1: working conditions, Factor 2: job stress and, Factor 3: work motivation and support. The work life items and associated factor loadings for each of the three factors are listed in Table 2.

To evaluate differences in practitioners' assessments of their work lives, an analysis of variance was carried out for each factor score (the loadings for all the items are included in factor scores). Significant differences between practitioner groups were found for two factors, "working conditions" (p < 0.05), and "job stress" (p < 0.01). The nurses view their working conditions and job stress less favorably than do HSWs. These two factors are discussed above, supported by the representative work-life items showing significant differences across practitioner group.

Table 3 reveals significant differences in the mean ratings from the two practitioner groups for each work-life variable. Significant (p < 0.05) t-values are printed in bold. The negative signs in the "Difference" and "t-value" columns of Table 3 reflect situations in which the mean rating for nurses exceeds that for HSWs. Large mean scores indicate a lower level of satisfaction with each item. Table 3 reveals significant differences in the mean ratings of all 22 work-life items across the two practitioner groups, while illustrating items that were not included in one of the three factors due to low loadings. The latter suggests that restructuring impacts upon all groups, particularly with both practitioner groups having negative responses to the items "pay is good" and "benefit package is good." This again reflects the

TABLE 2: Exploratory Factor Analysis Results for Work Life Item Loadings on Obliquely Rotated Factors

ITEM OBLIQUE ROTATED LOADINGS COMMON VARIANCES	FACTOR 1: WORKING CONDITIONS	FACTOR 2: JOB STRESS	FACTOR 3: MOTIVATION & SUPPORT
f) chances for promotion are good	**0.64**	-0.06	0.26
u) respected by community members	**0.50**	0.21	-0.16
d) job security is good	**0.44**	-0.05	0.04
k) enjoy commuting between clients	**0.43**	0.06	-0.07
t) hours are flexible & convenient	**0.42**	-0.20	-0.06
p) job responsibilities decreasing	0.01	**-0.61**	-0.02
o) job requires resourcefulness	0.06	**0.40**	-0.14
s) work is not stressful	0.12	**-0.40**	-0.27
j) have enough time to get job done	0.30	**-0.36**	-0.08
v) are not supervised too closely	-0.07	-0.11	**-0.56**
i) work is personally rewarding	-0.03	0.10	**-0.52**
l) are at ease in clients' homes	0.07	0.10	**-0.47**
e) enjoy clients	0.07	0.18	**-0.40**
g) respected by other members of the health-care team	0.15	-0.04	**-0.44**
c) good support from & communicate with office staff	0.10	-0.30	**-0.37**
q) employees are chosen fairly when extra work is available	-0.00	-0.20	**-0.35**

NOTE1: The factor loadings greater than 0.3 are in bold.
NOTE2: Items have been somewhat shortened from the original questionnaire version for space economy.
NOTE3: Six other work-life items not listed here were included in the analysis, but did not show loadings greater than 0.3 for any of the three factors.

disadvantaged position of home-care practitioners in the health-care hierarchy. Ten of the 22 work-life items differ significantly between the practitioner groups and help explain the results of the factor analysis.

TABLE 3: Differences Between Groups for Working Life Items

QUALITY OF WORK LIFE ITEMS	HSW MEANS	RN/RPN MEANS	DIFFER-ENCE	T-VALU E
a) work is interesting	**1.48**	**1.34**	**0.135**	**2.25**
b) pay is good	2.88	2.74	0.143	1.47
c) good support and communication with office staff (F3)	**1.90**	**2.32**	**-0.421**	**-3.77**
d) job security is good (F1)	2.10	2.28	-0.181	-1.80
e) enjoy clients (F3)	1.24	1.21	0.034	0.61
f) chances for promotion good (F1)	2.97	3.03	-0.058	-0.59
g) are respected by other members of health care team (F3)	1.96	1.87	0.084	0.79
h) a lot of freedom to decide how to do your work	2.02	1.97	0.043	0.47
i) work personally rewarding (F3)	**1.78**	**1.33**	**0.449**	**4.63**
j) have enough time to get job done (F2)	**1.85**	**2.29**	**-0.439**	**-5.07**
k) enjoy commuting between clients (F1)	2.07	1.95	0.124	1.21
l) at ease in clients' homes (F3)	**1.64**	**1.36**	**0.282**	**3.20**
m) are comfortable with medical equipment	1.65	1.63	0.027	0.36
n) benefit package is good	2.5	2.64	-0.137	-1.18
o) job requires resourcefulness (F2)	**1.56**	**1.21**	**0.351**	**6.72**
p) job responsibilities are decreasing (F2)	**3.13**	**3.64**	**-0.506**	**-6.61**
q) employees are chosen fairly when extra work is available (F3)	2.26	2.29	-0.034	-0.28
r) feel well-trained	**1.66**	**1.82**	**-0.198**	**-2.51**
s) work is not stressful (F2)	**2.75**	**3.07**	**-0.323**	**-3.65**
t) hours are flexible and convenient (F1)	**1.59**	**2.16**	**-0.565**	**-6.15**
u) respected by community members (F1)	1.61	1.58	0.028	0.38
v) not supervised too closely (F3)	1.72	1.76	-0.037	-0.44

NOTE1: Bolded items show a significant difference between practitioner groups, as the t-values are at or beyond the 0.05 level.
NOTE2: Items have been somewhat shortened from the original questionnaire for space economy.

Bibliography

Abel, E.K. & M.K. Nelson (eds.) (1990). *Circles of Care: Work and Identity*, Albany, State University of New York.

Alan, B. & C. Duncan (1990). *Quantitative Analysis for Social Scientists*, New York, Routledge.

Algoma District Health Council (1996). *Multi-Year Plan for Community Long-Term Care Services*, Sault Ste. Marie, Algoma District Health Council.

Armstrong, P., H. Armstrong, J. Choiniere, G. Feldberg, & J. White (1994). *Take Care: Warning Signals for Canada's Health System,* Toronto, Garamond.

Armstrong, P., J. Choiniere, E. Day (eds.) (1993). *Vital Signs: Nursing in Transition*, Toronto, Garamond.

Armstrong, P. & H. Armstrong (1990). *Theorizing Women's Work*. Toronto, Garamond Press.

Aronson, J. & S.M. Neysmith (1997). "The Retreat of the State and Long-Term Care Provision: Implications for Frail Elderly People, Unpaid Family Carers and Paid Home Care Workers," *Studies in Political Economy,* 53, 37-66.

Aronson, J. & S.M. Neysmith (1996). "'You're Not Just In There To Do The Work': Depersonalizing Policies and the Exploitation of Home Care Workers' Labour," *Gender & Society,* 10:1, 59-77.

Bakshi, P., M. Goodwin, J. Painter & A. Southern (1995). "Gender, Race and Class in the Local Welfare State: Moving Beyond Regulation Theory in Analyzing the Transition from Fordism," *Environment and Planning*, 27, 1555-1576.

Barnett, P. & R. Barnett (1997). "A Turning Tide? Reflections on Ideology and Health Service Restructuring in New Zealand," *Health & Place*, 3:1, 55-58.

Beggs, C. (1991). "Retention factors for Physiotherapists in an Underserviced Area: An Experience in Northern Ontario," *Physiotherapy Canada*, 43:2, 15-21.

Brief, A.P., R.S. Schuler & M. Van Sell (1981). *Managing Job Stress*, Boston, Little, Brown & Co.

Brodie, J. (1994). "Shifting the Boundaries: Gender and the Politics of Restructuring," in I. Bakker (ed.), *The Strategies of Silence: Gender and Economic Policy*, London, North-South Institute, 46-60.

Brown, P. & R. Scase (1991). *Poorwork: Disadvantage and the Division of Labour*, Philadelphia, PA, Open University Press.

Butter, I., E.Carpenter, B. Kay, & R. Simmons (1985). *Sex and Status: Hierarchies in the Health Workforce*, Washington, D.C., American Public Health Association.

Cameron, S.J., M.E. Horsburgh, & M. Armstrong-Stassen (1994). "Job Satisfaction, Propensity to Leave and Burnout in RNs and RNAs: A Multivariate Perspective," *Canadian Journal of Nursing Administration, 7*:3, 43-64.

Canadian Nurses Association & Canadian Hospital Association (1990). *Nurse Retention and Quality of Worklife: A National Perspective*, Ottawa, Canadian Nurses' Association.

Connelly, M.P. (1995). "Gender Matters: Restructuring and Adjustment, South and North," in *Gender and Economic Structuring*, Ontario, York University, Centre for Research on Work and Society, Working Paper Series No. 12.

Coutts, J. (1996). "Privatizing care for patients at home: an issue on the boil." *The Globe and Mail*, April 17, A8.

Dear, M., G. Clark, & S. Clark (1979). "Economic Cycles and Mental Health Care Policy: An Examination of the Macro-Context for Social Service Planning," *Social Science and Medicine, 13C*, 43-53.

Donovan, R. (1989). "Work Stress and Job Satisfaction: A Study of Home Care Workers in New York City," *Home Health Care Services Quarterly*, 10, 97-114.

Duffy, A. & N. Pupo (1992). *Part-time Paradox: Connecting Gender, Work and Family*, Toronto, McClelland & Stewart.

Duran-Arenas, L. & M. Lopez-Cervantes, M. (1996). "Health Care Reform and the Labour Market," *Social Science & Medicine*, 43:5, 791-797.

Employment and Immigration Canada (1989). *Workers with Family Responsibilities in a Changing Society: Who Cares?* Ottawa, Employment and Immigration Canada.

Esland, G., & G. Salaman (1980). *The Politics of Work & Occupations*, Toronto, University of Toronto Press.

Evans, P.M., & G.R. Wekerle (1997). *Women and the Canadian Welfare State: Challenges and Change*, Toronto, University of Toronto Press.

Fisher, B. (1990). "Alice in the Human Services: A Feminist Analysis of Women in the Caring Professions," in E.K. Abel & M.K. Nelson (eds.), *Circles of Care: Work and Identity in Women's Lives*, Albany, NY, State University of New York Press, 108-131.

Giddens, A. (1984). *The Constitution of Society: Outline of the Theory of Structuration*, Oxford, Polity Press.

Glazer, N. (1993). *Women's Paid and Unpaid Labour: The Work Transfer in Health Care and Retailing*, Philadelphia: Temple University Press.

Goldfarb Corporation (1988). *The Nursing Shortage in Ontario: A Research Report for the Ontario Nurses' Association*, Toronto, Ontario Nurses' Association.

Green, E., L. Hobbs & J. Mousseau (1994). "Introducing Quality Management in the Community: The VON Experience," *Canadian Journal of Nursing Administration*, 7:1, 62-75.

Gregson, N. & M. Lowe (1994). *Servicing the Middle Classes*, London, Routledge.

Hagerstrand, T. (1975). "Space, Time and Human Conditions," in A. Karlqvist, L. Lundqvist, and F. Snickars (eds.), *Dynamic Allocation of Urban Space*, Farnborough, Saxon House, 3-14.

Hanson, S. & G. Pratt (1995). *Gender, Work and Space*, London, Routledge.

Hudson, R. & T.A. Sullivan (1990). *The Social Organization of Work*, Belmont, CA, Wadsworth.

Hunter, D.J. (1996). "The Changing Roles of Health Care Personnel in Health and Health Care Management," *Social Science & Medicine*, 43:5, 799-808.

Hurst, J.W. (1991). "Reforming Health Care in Seven European Nations," *Health Policy*, 24:5, 7-14.

Janelle, D. (1969). "Spatial Reorganization: a Model and Concept," *Annals of the Association of American Geographers*, 59, 348-64.

Kearns, R. & J. Barnett (1992). "Enter the Supermarket: Entrepreneurial Medical Practice in New Zealand," *Environment and Planning C: Government Policy*, 10, 267-281.

Kim, J. & C.W. Mueller (1978). *Factor Analysis: Statistical Methods and Practical Issues*, Newbury Park, CA, Sage Publications.

Kobayashi, A., L. Peake, H. Benenson, & K. Pickles (1994). "Introduction: Placing Women and Work," in A. Kobayashi (ed.), *Women, Work, and Place*, Montreal/Kingston, McGill-Queen's University Press, xi-xiv.

Konka, J. (1995). Director, Home Care Program, Algoma Health Unit, Sault Ste. Marie. *Personal interview.*

Laws, G. (1989). "Deinstitutionalization and Privatization: Community-based Residential Care Facilities in Ontario," in J.L. Scarpaci (ed.), *Health Services Privatization in Industrial Societies,* New Brunswick, N.J., Rutgers University Press, 182-200.

Lee, R. (1991). *The Dictionary of Human Geography*, Oxford, Basil Blackwell.

Lesemann, F., & C. Martin (eds.) (1993). *Home-Based Care, The Elderly, The Family and The Welfare State: An International Comparison*, Ottawa, University of Ottawa Press.

Littler, C.R., & G. Salaman (1984). *Class at Work*, London, Batsford Academic & Educational Ltd.

Luxton, M. & E. Reiter (1997). "Double, Double, Toil and Trouble... Women's Experience of Work and Family in Canada, 1980-1995," in P.M. Evans & G.R. Wekerle (eds.), *Women and the Canadian Welfare State: Challenges and Change*, Toronto, University of Toronto Press, 198-221.

Massey, D. (1995). *Spatial Divisions of Labour*, Basingstoke, MacMillan.

McDowell, L. (1989). "Women in Thatcher's Britain," in *The Political Geography of Contemporary Britain*, Basingstoke, MacMillan.

McDowell, L. (ed.) (1994). *Defining Women: Social Institutions and Gender Divisions*, London, Polity Press.

Medjuck, S., M. O'Brien & C. Tozer (1992). "From Private Responsibility to Public Policy: Women and the Cost of Caregiving to Elderly Kin," *Atlantis: A Women's Studies Journal,* 17:2, 7-13.

Mohan, J. (1995). *A National Health Service? The Restructuring of Health Care in Britain since 1979,* New York, St. Martin's Press.

Monk, A. & C. Cox (1991). *Home Care for the Elderly: An International Perspective,* Westport, CT, Auburn House.

Ontario Ministry of Health (In-Home Services Branch) (1993). *Program Description: Placement Coordinator Services,* Ministry of Health, Ontario.

Oriol, W. (1985). *The Complex Cube of Long-Term Care,* Washington, D.C., American Health Planning Association.

Orloff, A. (1993). "Gender and the Social Rights of Citizenship: The Comparative Analysis of Gender Relations and Welfare States," *American Sociological Review,* 58:3, 303-28.

Peck, J. (1996). *Work Place: The Social Regulation of Labour Markets,* New York, Guilford.

Pinch, S. (1997). *Worlds of Welfare: Understanding the Changing Geographies of Social Welfare Provision,* London, Routledge.

Pines, A.M., E. Aronson & D. Karfrey (1981). *Burnout: From Tedium to Personal Growth,* New York, The Free Press.

Powell, M. (1995). "On the Outside Looking In: Medical Geography, Medical Geographers and Access to Health Care," *Health & Place,* 1:1, 41-50.

Price, J.L. (1994). "Total Quality Management Threatens Medicare," *Canadian Dimension,* Jan.-Feb., 15-20.

Rathwell, T. (1994). "Health Care in Canada: a System in Turmoil," *Health Policy,* 24, 5-17.

Richardson, T. (1994). *Patient-Focused Care: A United Nurses of Alberta Study,* Alberta, United Nurses of Alberta.

Richardson, T. (1993). *Total Quality Management Programs: More Work for Less Pay!* Alberta, United Nurses of Alberta.

Romero, M. (1994). "Chicanas and the Changing Work Experience in Domestic Service," in W. Giles & S. Arat-Koc (eds), *Maid in the Market*, Halifax, Fernwood Publishing, 48-55.

Rose, G. (1993). *Feminism and Geography: The Limits of Geographical Knowledge*, Cambridge, Polity Press.

Sacks, K.B. (1990). *Caring by the Hour: Women, Work and Organizing at Duke Medical Center*, Urbana, University of Illinois Press.

Sheppard, E & T. Barnes (1990). *The Capitalist Space Economy*, London, Unwin Hyman.

Sky, L. (1995). *Lean and Mean Health Care: The Creation of the Generic Worker and the Deregulation of Health Care*, Don Mills, Ontario Federation of Labour.

Tatroff, D. (1995). "Under the knife in Chilliwack: An American health care program rides into town," *Our Times*, 14:2, 14-38.

Thrift, N. & P. Williams (1987). *Class and Space: The Making of Urban Society*, London, Routledge and Kegan Paul.

Trade Union Research Bureau (1994). "Patient-focused Care: Hospital Re-engineering and the Union Response: Final Report," Commissioned by British Columbia Nurses' Union, Health Sciences Association of British Columbia, and Hospital Employees' Union, Vancouver.

Twaddle, A.C. (1996). "Health System Reforms—Toward a Framework for International Comparisons," *Social Science & Medicine*, 43:5, 637-654.

Van De Ven, W.P.M. (1996). "Market-Oriented Health Care Reform: Trends and Future Options," *Social Science & Medicine*, 43:5, 655-666.

Walker, R. (1985). "Class, Division of Labour and Employment in Space," in D. Gregory & J. Urry (eds.), *Social Relations and Spatial Structures*, New York, St. Martin's Press.

Webster, B. (1985). "A woman's issue: the impact of local authority cuts," *Local Government Studies*, 11, 19-46.

White, J. (1990). *Hospital Strike: Women, Unions, and Public Sector Conflict*, Toronto, Thompson Educational Publishing.

White, G. (1994). Personal correspondence. Ministry of Health (In-Home Care Branch), Toronto, Ontario.

Williams, A.M. (1996). "The History of Home Care in Ontario: A Geographical Analysis," *Social Science & Medicine*, 42:6, 937-948.

Notes

[1] I would like to thank the practitioner respondents and the two non-profit home-care organizations, without whom this work would not have been carried out. The guidance of Valerie Preston was essential to the completion of this work and I am greatly indebted to her for it. Parts of this chapter first appeared in different form in *Geographies of Women's Health* (London, Routledge, 2001, pp. 107-126), edited by I. Dyck, N. Lewis, and S. McLafferty. Thanks to the editors and to Taylor & Francis Books Limited, UK, for their permission to reproduce those sections.

[2] The methodology used in this case study is described in detail in the appendix to this chapter.

[3] It is the cumulative effect of the differences in the ratings of all items making up the factor "working conditions" that makes a significant difference between nurses and HSWs in the mean scores on this factor. Mean ratings between the two practitioner groups differ significantly on only one of the five items that load highly on this factor, "hours are flexible and convenient." Nurses have significantly ($p < 0.05$) lower overall levels of agreement (mean=2.16) with this statement than HSWs (mean=1.59).

Chapter 4
Offloading the Cost of Home Care: The Impact on Front-Line Workers and Agencies[1]
Denise O'Connor

1. Introduction

After its election in 1995, the Harris government approached health-care reform with the attitude that the system was broken on a number of fronts. This feeling was informed by a national and international neoliberal discourse that repeated three fundamental ideas. These were:
1. that growing, ageing populations will bankrupt public health systems;
2. that health systems everywhere need reform and that the best way to proceed is to introduce market mechanisms (Armstrong et al., 2000); and
3. that health-care costs are spiraling out of control.

In the early and mid-1990s, Ontario governments were faced with the largest budget deficits in the province's history. The fiscal challenge was exacerbated by the impact of reduced federal transfer payments. The federal government repeatedly reduced its transfers to the provinces under the Canada Assistance Plan and Established Programs Financing, its biggest cut coming in the 1995 federal budget, a few months before the Harris government's accession to power with a mandate to balance its budget within five years, while simultaneously reducing personal and corporate taxes. With pressures on both the revenue and cost sides, restructuring health care, the largest expenditure item in the provincial budget, became an important project for the Harris government.

In 1995, Ontario's home-care "system" was a "patchwork" of 36 placement co-ordinators and 38 home-care programs with different rules and different agreements across the province. Governments had essentially relegated the task of managing home care to the voluntary or third sector, consistent with their practices in other sectors of health care, education and social services. In that system, relationships were based on trust and embodied a spirit of collaboration. In a number of cases, a non-governmental organization, the Victorian Order of Nurses (VON), not only delivered services of its own, but co-ordinated home-care services more generally. However, this practice of both coordinating and delivering service violated one of the basic tenets of New Public Management, the separation of provision from production. The Harris government considered this to be particularly problematic in administrative terms: in being entirely managed by the third sector, home care lacked the normal accountability mechanisms that are built into more conventional public service arrangements. Former Premier Harris's testimony at Justice O'Connor's Inquiry on Tainted Water in Walkerton revealed the extent to which he believes that institutional actors' motivation is their own bureaucratic self-interest[2].

In 1996, the Ontario government announced that it was implementing a model of "managed competition" in the provision of home-care services and that this system would be managed by forty-three Community Care Access Centres (CCACs), non-profit agencies governed by local boards of directors. Managed competition represented an effort to introduce market mechanisms, namely competition, into what the government perceived to be an inefficient, self-serving home-care system managed by the third sector. Managed competition is the creation of a quasi-market through the deployment of a contracting process that theoretically will result in a more efficient allocation of resources. It involves the separation of provision (funding and assessing needs) from production (actual care and services). The CCAC, as the contracting body, functions as a proxy for the "consumer," or client, ascertaining the most efficient trade-off between quality and price, as measured during the proposal evaluation phase (Request for Proposal or RFP). This vision is premised on the notion that the CCAC, as a neutral body responsive to community needs, and thus without a vested interest in a particular outcome other than the best quality-cost trade-off, will provide a cost-efficient way of managing home-support services.

On February 1997, Health Minister Jim Wilson stated in the Ontario legislature: "We're getting rid of the empires of the past and replacing them with streamlined efficient delivery systems." Competition would slim home care down. In a market environment, wage rates would find their natural (read: lower) rate. This valuing of competition was coupled with a belief that the private sector is inherently more efficient than either the public or third sectors. Adoption of the new model created a "level playing field" by putting an end to the preference for the not-for-profit sector that had been the policy of previous administrations. This represented a fundamental shift in the relationship between the government and the third sector in Ontario. In essence, voluntary agencies were now treated like profit-seeking enterprises and were presumed to be acting to maximize their self-interest. Both Canadian and American for-profit firms were invited to compete for contracts. Managed competition was phased in over a four-year period that has now been completed. All home-support services have been tendered and all surviving provider agencies are operating under a contractual arrangement with their local CCAC.

Home care entails the direct provision of a human service to acutely ill or chronically debilitated clients in their homes. It is estimated that eighty per cent of the cost of delivering home care[3] is direct labour. (RNAO, 1999, 5) The remaining twenty percent supports front-line service through administrative and supervisory functions and some office overhead.[4] Invariably, any efforts to find "savings" will be directed necessarily at increasing productivity and/or reducing direct labour costs. As there is little or no technology involved in such human services, and it is not viable to substitute machinery for people (the conventional way of improving productivity), efforts at reducing costs centre on reducing or containing the cost of labour. In home care, "doing more with less"—one of the credos of public service reform—means working harder for less money.

The government of Ontario has attempted to control the costs of home care by creating a rigid institutional structure that entrenches its power, but has resulted in the disempowerment of both the organizations charged with implementing the policy as well as the front-line workers who have lost the discretion to respond to clients' needs as they arise. Three fundamental features underpin this reform:

1. price control;
2. narrowly defining home-care services and removing the discretion of front line workers to define the work; and
3. the introduction of competitive bidding.

Prices, at least in the initial round of contracts, were fixed over the period of the contract. Any increases in the cost of doing business had to have been anticipated and built into the three- or four-year price guaranteed to CCACs for service delivery at the *beginning* of a contract—price escalations were typically not permitted. Given the labour-intensive nature of the sector, this had a significant impact on compensation and employment conditions. It contributed to a human-resources crisis that emerged while home-care services were expanding. An unprecedented number of workers chose to reject these terms of employment and exit the sector. The Ontario Community Support Association, an association of the non-profit providers, estimated that the attrition rate for some providers ranges from 25 percent to 40 percent annually. (OCSA, 2000) The Ontario Association of CCACs reported that the Ottawa-Carleton CCAC had found the following attrition rates among nursing agencies: from a low of 20 percent to a high in one case of 75 percent for RNs, and a range of 16 to 61 percent for RPNs. (OACCAC, 2000) Those who left went to work in the hospital sector primarily. In Brant-Haldimand-Norfolk, over a one-year period the VON recorded a turnover rate of 29 percent for RNs and 27 percent for RPNs. Forty percent of the RNs went to work in the hospital sector.

The second feature is a narrowing of the definition of what appropriately constitutes fundable home-care services. The Long-term Care Regulations (implemented in 1999) are based on estimates of the standard amount of time required per home-care visit. No cost adjustment is made for visits that take longer than the allocated average. This represents a reduction of services to their technical parts, ignoring the role of interpersonal dynamics in providing such personal human services. It is, in essence, "taylorized" or assembly-line home care (see Browne in this volume).

The third feature is the fragmentation of the home-care sector through the introduction of competition, which affected both agencies and workers. Agencies that traditionally worked together in sharing experiences and best practices were pitted against each other and against for-profit firms in the competitive contracting process. "Best practices" were transformed into "competitive advantages" to be protected, not shared. Workers were disciplined by the implicit threat that they could be replaced legally should they seek better working conditions or compensation by taking labour action. Other agencies or suppliers were waiting in the wings and could do "their" work. The CCAC controls the flow of work and can divert it to whomever it chooses. Employment has effectively been uncoupled from the continuous supply of service.

2. CCACs: Managing Home Care Locally

The CCAC plays three roles: awarding contracts, case management, and managing the local home-care budget. Each of the forty-three CCACs decides the proportion of services allocated among RNs, Personal Support Workers (PSWs) and Home Support Workers (HSWs) (RNAO, 1999) in response to what it identifies as its community's needs. CCAC budgets come from the Ministry of Health and Long-Term Care (MOHLTC). The parameters of service provision are described by a series of regulations that dictate what services are to be paid for and the limitations on the service mix and frequency of visits per client. (Assistant Deputy Minister, 1999) CCACs have a very narrow, highly defined mandate. The Ministry exercises a high level of control over the services the CCACs can provide, and the latter, in turn, do the same with the provider agencies. Additionally, CCACs are required to develop an annual business plan submitted for approval to their local MOHLTC office. Annual budgets are capped. Under the previous system, budgets were viewed as guidelines, but the system was driven by local demand and governments covered deficits. Now CCACs are required to work within their budgets and ration service accordingly. The case managers, who provide the interface between patient intake and the service agency, are charged with rationing these services. (Broadcast News, 2001)

Waiting lists are permitted for all services but nursing. (OACCAC, 2000) Thus, the balance of services are to be rationed through the use of waiting lists (RNAO, 1999), with cost containment marking the cut-off point for service. There has been a reduction in services to the frail elderly, children with complex needs and adults with long-term disabilities. (RNAO, 1999) Acute-care patients have displaced them. By definition, acutely ill patients have priority over non-acute patients, nursing services are considered critical, and service must be provided immediately. But labour-market shortages that occurred even before the 2001 budget caps have meant that there have, in fact, been waiting lists. The Ontario Association of CCACs (OACCAC) reported that the four nursing agencies under contract with the Toronto CCAC were "unable to service" 183 times in the first three months of the year 2000, affecting 70 clients. These include services such as changing wound dressings or analyzing diabetics' blood sugar. The failure to provide service resulted in some patients remaining in hospital or being referred to walk-in clinics or Emergency Rooms for treatment. This ended up costing the system more money. In some cases, patients had to return in dire circumstances to the Emergency Room, because they had not received adequate care in the community. These incidents have been directly attributed to the human-resources crisis (RNAO, 1999) that occurred when home care was expanding, but wages remained static.

CCACs were originally incorporated as non-profit organizations, accountable to the community through boards of directors elected by their members and charged with managing the home care system in their region. In February 2002, they were converted to statutory agencies under the Community Care Access Corporations Act (2002). Henceforth, their boards of directors are appointed by Order-in-Council. As non-profit community organizations, CCACs had little influence on government policy, but were at least theoretically "independent" of government. However, they were becoming increasingly vocal in identifying the shortfall in government funding of the home-care

The Commodity of Care   153

sector, particularly in the wake of the May 2001 provincial budget, and had taken their concerns directly to the public through the media. Rather than address the funding issues, the Harris government put an end to dissent. Cabinet appointees have replaced many boards and chief executive officers (the *Kingston Whig Standard* reported that local Conservative riding associations were asked to compile lists of candidates to sit on CCAC boards for consideration by the Ministry [Lukits, 2002]). CCACs are no longer directly accountable to their local community. They are directly answerable only to cabinet.

3. Contracting with Service Providers

Each CCAC has entered into contractual agreements with service providers who employ the appropriate staff. Separate contracts for fixed periods are awarded for each type of service: nursing, homemaking, professional therapy and so forth. The timing of these contracts is staggered. On the market model, each of these services was to be divided among a number of providers to increase the flexibility of the system and presumably to decrease the bargaining power of the agencies and of their employees. This was more easily accomplished in urban than rural areas, because there was not sufficient business to attract a range of providers in the latter. (O'Connor, 1999) Contracts are awarded for market share, with no guarantee of volume levels. This permits the government to increase or decrease local budgets with impunity.

Workers were expected to move with the work, once contracts began to be awarded under the new system. Yet, when Saint-Elizabeth Nursing closed its homemaking operation in Hamilton, only about 40 of its 128 workers moved to the remaining non-profit agency. (OCSA, 2000) Eighty-eight trained workers left the sector. Thus, the transition in providers can result in both instability and loss of labour capacity. Exit interviews performed by one provider suggested that workers typically move to the more stable institutional sector, or leave the sector completely—taking jobs in retail or even in abattoirs, where the conditions are more stable and predictable (interview with agency expert, May 2001).

Under the previous system, preference for not-for-profit providers was written into the law, which meant that non-profit organizations got the majority of client referrals. The for-profit sector also received referrals under this system. They would get the evening and weekend work, which non-profit organizations were not interested in providing (interview with expert in for-profit sector, November 1999). There were wage disparities between the two sectors, with the non-profit organizations offering better pay and benefits to their employees, and the for-profits offering part-time casual employment with few or no benefits.

Contracts are now open to both the for-profit sector and non-profit organizations. Agencies compete with each other on the basis of a price/quality mix that is ascertained by each CCAC to offer the best value. In order to compete with the for-profit sector, non-profit organizations reduced their compensation and benefit packages. (HDHC, 2000) Many employers have replaced full-time with part-time, casual employees, to meet the flexibility requirements of the CCAC.

The CCAC pays for nursing and homemaking services on a per visit basis. (RNAO, 1999) Some contracts include penalties that allow CCACs to fine agencies when they are unable to take a referral for any reason. If a procedure takes longer than scheduled, the agency, and in turn the worker, are not paid for that extra time. However, in emergencies a call can be made to the CCAC and an extension be negotiated and approved (interview with agency expert, April 28, 2002). The Hamilton District Health Council reports that "home care agency fiscal pressures are being felt by home care's direct care workers who report having to perform extra hours of unpaid work due to the minimal level of time assessed to complete required tasks." (HDHC, 2001) Home-care workers are faced with the choice of leaving a client in a precarious situation—which is really not a choice at all, particularly in view of the moral and legal dimensions of such a course of action—or working for free. Because home care is essentially constructed as piecework, work that does not fit into the government's definition of what is to be done, or that exceeds the estimated time required to perform them, is offloaded onto workers and agencies by the government and its agent, the CCAC (see Browne in this volume).

The CCACs do not pay for the time it takes home-care workers to travel from one client to another, yet agencies are required to compensate their employees for it in accordance with employment standards (interviews with agency experts April 28, 2002 and May 2001). A few offer a mileage rate to offset expenses, again not compensated by the CCAC. This is complicated further by the fact that the duration of visits has shortened over the period of the reforms. Every worker now sees more clients, but for a shorter time each, thus getting fewer continuous hours of "work" and increasing the employer's portion of wages that are not reimbursed by the unit fee (interview with agency experts, April 28, 2002, and May 2001). This creates a tension between clients', workers', and agencies' needs. Clients may want the same worker at a certain time each day, but this will serve as a constraint on optimal scheduling. Some agencies have developed strategies to organize workers' time more efficiently by realigning their workforce into neighbourhood teams and some CCACs cooperate with this effort by allowing the agency to build its schedules around workers' timetables rather than clients'. Other CCACs insist that priority must be given to clients' preferences, rather than to an "efficient" organization of workers' time.

A single patient can have a number of home-care workers coming from different agencies to provide an array of support services. The case manager, who is employed by the CCAC, is charged with coordinating these services. Service providers do not necessarily consult with one another and may not even know who else is providing service to the client. They are unlikely to be from the same organization. Many case managers are RNs, but social workers have also been hired to fill that role. (RNAO, 1999) This can occasion tension between frontline RNs and case workers. This tension is compounded by the power imbalance. While the case manager has the full weight of government authority behind her, the agency supervisor or worker may be viewed only as a contracted technician, acting to maximize her organization's revenue base. This dynamic reduces the likelihood of cooperative problem solving.

4. The Impact of Managed Competition on Non-Profit Agencies

The new system of managed competition brought enormous change to Ontario's home-care sector. However, it was very much an imposed process and was imperfectly conceived. Serious pathologies emerge when organizations are unresponsive to change. In home care, all actors will react with short-term survival strategies when health rationing and cost-containment strategies collide with this model of managed competition.

In a competitive environment, agencies will work collaboratively with other providers to promote the interests of the sector and their clients, but not at the expense of ensuring their own continued viability and retaining their competitive advantage. The sharing of best practices has diminished as a result of this. Prior to managed competition, the non-profit sector had a culture of sharing information with other agencies, leading to best practices and emulation of innovative initiatives. Now such knowledge and expertise is protected as a competitive advantage. Non-profit service providers speak of this as a very negative effect of managed competition (interviews with agency experts, November 1999, May 2001, June 2001), which is at odds with all of the conventional wisdom of experts in health and social service provision.

Providers have also had difficulty in working within the fiscal constraints of a price frozen for three to four years. Consequently, a number of agencies have attempted to reopen contracts. This occurs at the discretion of the CCAC, with some CCACs being more receptive to this overture than others. Unable to absorb increased costs, and with no opportunity to pass them along, agencies have been forced into bankruptcy. An inordinate amount of time and energy is spent managing crises, rather than engaging in productive endeavours (interviews with agency experts, May 2001, personal experience as a board member). Coupled with a cost-containment strategy, managed competition has created volatility and instability in home care.

Home-care delivery requires more than negotiating a simple set of straightforward, technical services—easily delivered, measured, evaluated. Public policy must be implemented effectively. Leslie Pal characterizes successful implementation as a combination of "top-down" and "bottom-up processes" that "take place in a world of multiple powers and authorities, organizations, and personalities." (Pal, 1997) An environment of collaboration and cooperation is necessary to increase the chances of successful implementation. Policy makers must learn from those who deliver services, in order to increase the effectiveness of public policies.

However, in the case of home care, how the policy process unfolds is very much in the hands of government authorities. The agencies that employ the front-line workers have very little power or influence. They are twice removed from the primary funder, the provincial government, and are limited to negotiating with the government's agents—the Community Care Access Centres. The government has also shown little interest in the CCACs' experience, as it demonstrated by converting them into statutory agencies when they dared to speak out. This becomes problematic when implementation problems, such as the human resources shortage, emerge. The CCACs had neither the authority, nor the fiscal capacity, to deal with the problem.

5. Labour Markets and the Delivery of Public Goods

Labour market theories typically focus on the private sector where market mechanisms are at play. As such, notions of how labour markets function may offer valuable insights and models, but have limited application in the area of government provision when it comes to negotiating wage rates.

The "market" for public goods is governed by a different logic than that of private goods. Demand for health care, education, and the like is driven by demography, need, and citizens' expectations—and, of course, governments' ability and willingness to pay. "Consumption" of some goods, such as health care and education, is not discretionary in the traditional sense of the word. Demand responds to a logic that is separate from the logic of supply. Supply is limited by governments' willingness to provide services, but supply problems can also be exacerbated by labour shortages. Shortages of supply can become manifest, for example, as waiting lists for surgical procedures, occurrences of emergency room by-pass, or a shortage of diagnostic equipment. These become potent public symbols of a system in "crisis." What is less visible and measurable—and more easily obfuscated— is the effect of labour markets and the degree to which these are artificial constructs.

In the production of public goods, demand and supply are both tied to a given place. In the eyes of some, this dynamic coupled with government "monopoly" provision led to exorbitant wages for public employees during the expansion of the welfare state. Public servants have been characterized as poor producers and profligate, while governments have been accused of systematically wasting "taxpayers' dollars." The response to this perceived problem has been to discipline the labour market by means by rationing resources, i.e., by imposing budgetary austerity. Workers have been admonished to "do more with less."

Government policy determines the structure of the interactions within the public-sector "labour market." Legal power and authority to design and implement policy rests with the government. It has the power to decide whether to negotiate directly with workers providing public goods or to relegate this task to a third party.

In the health-care sector, wage negotiations occur both directly and indirectly with government. Doctors negotiate directly with the Ministry of Health and Long-Term Care (MOHLTC) through their professional organization, as do hospital nurses. Other hospital workers negotiate with their hospitals. Hospitals receive global budgets from the MOHLTC. They consequently have some discretion to decide how to allocate resources within their institution. (Haiven, 1995) The extent to which workers can wield their collective power depends on such factors as unionization rates, their strength and cohesion as a sector, and how easily and effectively workers are replaceable.

Home care is a highly fragmented labour sector, as workers negotiate only with their direct employer. In most communities, contracts have been divided among three to five agencies. Home-care agencies, in turn, sign contracts with the CCAC on a fee-for-service basis. This means they are funded only for delivering a specific service on a competitive basis with other agencies. The CCAC is, of course, funded by the MOHLTC.

Home-care workers are thus twice-removed from the funder and their employers' revenues are entirely dependent on demand, directly linked to, and limited by, the volume of service they provide. The agencies cannot store their products in inventory. An hour lost is lost forever. This may be ideal from the perspective of the funder, but can wreak havoc with workers and agencies. Workers cannot predict their pay cheques from one week to the next. Agencies must manage their fixed costs in a very uncertain environment.

Nowhere but in public provision are markets more clearly socially and culturally constructed with the only "pure" economic variable in place being the *opportunity cost* of labour; that is what their labour is worth when sold elsewhere. Workers are not necessarily confined to working in the labour markets for public goods. If their skills are transferable and better compensated in the private sector they have the choice to sell their labour in that sector. Thus, there is leakage between the two sectors when it comes to labour. This affects both retention rates in each sector and the capacity of each sector to attract employees. Moreover, it has an effect on expectations for compensation. This creates a tension between what labour wants and what governments are prepared to pay. The power that this represents varies with the labour supply. Traditionally, this means that when labour is in short supply, labour should be able to command higher wages. However, funding service through rigid contracts reduces the flexibility in the employer-employee relationship and decreases the responsiveness of organizations to emergent conditions. The result, in the case of home care, is that organizations become uncompetitive and suffer labour shortages when they lack the fiscal flexibility to respond to changing labour conditions.

An OACCAC report written at the height of the human resources crisis, sees a major problem in the "lack of competitiveness of the community care sector, not only with other areas of health care, but also other broader public and private sector employment opportunities with respect to compensation and working conditions." It adds that there are "competing educational and career opportunities for

women who have traditionally chosen careers in health care."
(OACCAC, 2000) When women have choices, fewer are choosing to
work in this sector.

6. Stratification of Workers

Within the home care sector there is a stratification of workers. At the
top are registered nurses (RNs), professionals who are college or university trained and governed by a professional college. Next are the
personal support workers (PSWs), who are college trained (private or
public). Their duties include personal care tasks, which includes bathing and other such personal tasks, in addition to the tasks assigned
Home Support Workers (HSWs). The latter, traditionally, do not
require any formal training, but may have an "interest in gerontology,
excellent interpersonal, organizational and communication skills, the
ability to work independently and a physical ability to perform
housecleaning. HSWs provide emotional support, housekeeping tasks,
meal preparation, laundry, shopping, banking, activation assistance,
housecleaning and other unspecified duties."[5] Homemaking agencies
themselves are stratified. Supervisors are primarily registered nurses.
This sets a limit on the career path of HSWs and PSWs.

Almost every front-line worker in this labour market is female.
Moreover, Zeytinoglu and Muteshi cite a number of Canadian studies that show that "[w]hite women were more likely to be in the core,
skilled jobs of visiting nurses and therapists, while racial minority
women were employed in the peripheral, lesser skilled jobs of home
support workers." (Zeytinoglu, 2000) In other words, this labour
market is both gendered and racialized.

There has been a shift in who does what over the last six or seven
years. Tasks such as bathing, catheterizing patients, and teaching exercise regimes, which were the purview of nurses, are now done by PSWs
(interviews with agency experts November 1999 and May 2001). In
the public and political discourse home care is typically identified as
nursing services, rendering PSWs and HSWs invisible in the public
and political consciousness despite the fact that they command the
greatest share of hours of service provided. The Ontario Association

for CCACs reports that the Ministry of Health and Long Term Care shows an 18 percent increase in the number of clients served between 1996-97 and 1997-98. The OACCAC demonstrates that a comparison of 1994-95 and 1997-98 shows there was a 31 percent increase in nursing visits (1,606,000) and a 25 percent increase in homemaking hours (3,780,000). (OACCAC, 2000) These data also reveal that homemaking hours significantly exceed those of nursing. Browne identifies an increase in nursing visits of 30.8 percent between 1997-1999 and 24.9 percent in homemaking for a similar period. (Browne, 2000) An Ontario Home Health Providers Association and Ontario Community Support Association (the industry associations for the for-profit and NPO sectors respectively) report that funding to CCACs increased 21 percent from 1998 to 2000/01. (OHHCPA & OCSA, 2001) Increases of this magnitude typically occurred because CCAC spending exceeded their budget allocations. In the 2001/02 budget, there was no increase and it has been made clear the CCACs that deficits will not be tolerated. Stripping away their independence has assured the government of that.

Hospitals are discharging patients "quicker and sicker" with the result that there has been an increase in the acuity of patients cared for in the community. Nurses argue that this double shift (who does what and where) compromises the quality of patient care. They have argued, for example, when bathing a patient an RN would also be doing a general health check that a less skilled worker cannot. Similarly, having PSWs catheterize patients poses the same type of risks. A study conducted for Human Resources Development Canada suggests that the increase in the acuity of clients in the community requires higher levels of initial training for unregulated workers as well as access to on-going training. Typically, however, the cost of training has been offloaded to workers. This is problematic because most simply cannot afford to exchange unpaid training time for paid work hours, if they are even able to schedule the time in their irregular day. (HRDC, 2001) Moreover, there is no mandatory requirement in Ontario that continuing education be done, while home-care contracts make no distinction between agencies that provide training and agencies that do not.

7. Dynamics Across the Health Sectors: Comparing Work Conditions

RNs, of course, can also work in the hospital sector and the institutional long-term care sector. Wages for RNs in the community sector range from $16 to $23 per hour and in the hospital sector from $20.50 to $30.25. (RNAO, 1999) Furthermore, community-based RNs travel from client to client. Travel time is not paid at the full hourly rate, it is negotiated between each agency and its workers. Similarly, PSWs and HSWs either need a car or timely and reliable access to public transit to travel between clients. Prior to the VON strike in Hamilton in September, 2000, VON Hamilton nurses were paid 15¢ per kilometer for car expenses, compared to the standard set by the Auditor-General in tax assessment of 28¢ - 30¢. This was changed in VON's strike-settling collective agreement (interview with agency expert, May 2001).

Community RNs may not be guaranteed a set number of hours of work on even a weekly basis, let alone daily. In the hospital sector a nurse is guaranteed at least four consecutive hours of work for a shift. In the community, if a client cancels, the worker may or may not be sent somewhere else. Agencies are not typically reimbursed by their CCAC for cancelled visits, which means not only lost wages for the worker, but that administrative costs for the agencies are not recovered.

Similarly PSWs[6] can work in both the community and long-term care institutional sector. In Hamilton, for example, the disparity in wages ranges from $5.00 to $6.00 per hour. (HDHC, 2000) As is the case with nurses, in the institutional sector a PSW would be guaranteed at least four consecutive hours of work, and more likely eight or twelve. The MOHLTC budgets for higher wages for institutional workers in its funding formula.

8. The Nature of the Work

Home-care workers are, in essence, guests in other people's homes. They work in isolation from colleagues and rarely have on-site supervision or support. Aronson and Neysmith (1999) describe them as "a labour force of low paid para-professionals, drawn increasingly from immigrant populations in a metropolitan areas, who do what is understood in our culture as the ordinary activities of women in the privacy of old people's homes." They point to the literature on institutional work to highlight the conceptualization of the work of home-care workers by the public and governments. Factors largely ignored, or the import of which is minimized, include:

the complexity and invisibility of the emotional work involved in caring for people's personal needs; the poor employment conditions and devalued status of nursing assistants and aides who are key care providers for chronically ill and frail elderly people; and the negative effects of managerial practices that seek to cut government costs by intensifying and pressing the caring labour process into the standardized form of industrial production. (Aronson & Neysmith, 1999)

Caring work is, to reiterate the point, an invisible part of the job. Aronson and Neysmith describe a "significant discrepancy" between workers' official job descriptions and their own accounts of what they do. An important part of the job, according to workers, is the ability to individualize their relationship to meet their clients' needs: "home-care workers prided themselves on their ability to personalize their work in this way, on building relationships and on caring well for their clients. The attachment they developed with clients is an inevitable and, often, rewarding aspect of their job." (Aronson & Neysmith, 1999)

Aronson and Neysmith (1999) further point out that home-care workers are exploited by the system: "workers described various ways in which their work seeped out its formal boundaries. For example, they put in time beyond their official allocation of hours [and] ... carried out tasks that lay outside their officially defined repertoire .... which they judged would benefit their elderly clients." The motivation for this behaviour was a moral obligation to help the vulnerable; but it was "also extracted by virtue of home-care workers' vulnerable social status. This vulnerability originated, for them all, in their status as workers deemed relatively unskilled and easily replaceable." As one worker succinctly put it "if I don't have them [my clients] I don't work. I don't have pay. And I need my pay to eat."

The work done with patients has been reduced to its technical components, or taylorized, through the process of health care restructuring. According to the RNAO, "nurses report that case managers: require care plans that focus on nursing tasks and do not address the holistic needs, such as education and psychosocial needs of clients and their families; approach care-plan development solely from a cost-control perspective." Hence what workers regard as critically important to the job is neither compensated, nor recognized as important. Workers have little discretion in determining their patients' needs. The RNAO concludes that "the focus of both CCACs and providers has shifted from 'quality care for all clients' to a 'bottom line' approach." (RNAO, 1999)

A majority of workers deplore their lack of control over their jobs and feel disheartened by the unpredictability of their working hours. (Denton et al., 1999) Workers do not always feel that supervisors are sufficiently concerned about their safety.

> There was one fellow who was, uh, an ex-con. It was like something out of a movie—run-down building and back doors, and you never know. You don't know what you don't need to and that's the bottom line. Actually at first I didn't know [that he was an ex-con]. I'd been going two or three times. I was in the office, it wasn't brought up. I don't know. I breezed right in there. I didn't know until a few days later what his background was. It just wasn't thought to be an important piece of information, I guess. (Denton et al., 2000)

Agencies have to balance an employee's right to work in safety with clients' rights to their own preferences. For example, agencies are confronted with legal and ethical dilemmas when they are asked to send only white workers, as sometimes happens. Nonetheless, many home-support workers report a great deal of job satisfaction, due mainly to the positive relationships they forge with their clients. (Denton et al.,

The Commodity of Care 165

1999) It is worth noting, however, that studies indicating this were done prior to the reforms.

To conclude, it is difficult for home-support workers to earn a decent living within a reasonably contained workday in this sector. Moreover, the career paths of personal-support workers and home-makers are limited. It does not get any better than a long, unpredictable day at low wages. Little wonder that other sectors provide an attractive alternative.

9. Power Relations

CCACs are designed to arrange the delivery of a specific basket of public goods in a narrowly prescribed way. They serve as a buffer between government and the agencies that implement public policy by providing these goods. The lack of discretion afforded CCACs in policy implementation has a direct effect on home-care agencies and this is compounded by the reality of the competitive model. For agencies and workers, the threat of being replaced is omnipresent. By parcelling work out among a number of agencies in each community, the CCACs have the option of moving business around if agencies are unable to accommodate their demands.

Workers have little bargaining power with their agencies, because agencies are vulnerable if labour action is undertaken. Strikes have resulted in agencies losing business, laying off employees, or even closing. (Huang, 2000; RNAO, 1999) With the opportunity to "voice" their concerns reduced, workers are left with the choice to "exit" the sector. Some workers are better positioned than others to exercise this exit option. Zeytinoglu et al. (2000) situate the treatment of this labour force within the context of an international trend in late capitalism to exploit women's work, and particularly that of non-white women, through the shift to flexible, casualized and part-time labour. In the racialized, gendered work force, white women typically holding the professional and supervisory roles and immigrant women the "less skilled" occupations.

This represents a heavy-handed, top-down approach to policy implementation. The government sets the budget and charges its local agents, the CCACs, with making the system work. There is little opportunity, it seems, for policy-learning to influence processes. This creates a problematic disjuncture between the policy-development and implementation processes. It reduces the system's responsiveness. Both the CCACs and the home-care agencies are forced to limp along with a poorly designed system.

10. Conclusion

In its effort to control the cost of home care through the introduction of competition, the government of Ontario has succeeded in created an unstable, volatile environment for both agencies and their workers. How can agencies manage their "businesses" when costs are unpredictable, because volumes are uncertain and patient acuity is increasing, yet revenues are limited by contractually fixed prices over an extended period of time? Given their high attrition rates, how can agencies ensure continuous quality when they are not compensated for ensuring their workers have continuous education? The horizon of their planning cycle is the next contract and they have but one goal: to ensure that they are positioned to be competitive in tendering for that contract. If they fail to get the contract they will in effect be shut out of the public home-care market. This creates a perverse incentive structure.

Workers face uncertainty on a weekly basis. How many hours will they work and where? Moreover, they must negotiate their terms of employment with employers who have very little room to manoeuvre, knowing that another agency can provide their services in the event of a strike. They have to ask themselves whether they can live with this level of unpredictability and the obviously poor prospects for improving their standard of living.

The government of Ontario, for its part, has distanced itself from answering for these problems by the creation of arm's-length statutory agencies, charged with managing this system within a very narrow set of parameters. One must wonder at what point the damage becomes irreparable.

Appendix: Methodology

This paper relied on a number of secondary sources as well as interviews conducted over the last three years as the author completed her graduate course work at McMaster University. Interviews were conducted at various times with agency Supervisors, Executive Directors, and CEOs (former and current) of both local and national organizations, and experts in industry associations of both the for-profit and non-profit sectors. Additionally, the author has served on the board of directors of a non-profit home-care provider for six years. This latter experience has provided a front-row seat in watching the impact of this new model and the unfolding of more recent events. Much of what is written here relies on her understanding of this sector through continuous probing and questioning of people working within it.

Bibliography

Broadcast News (2001). "Government moves to strengthen Community Care Access Centres," Toronto.

Armstrong, Pat et al. (2000). *Heal Thyself: Managing Health Care Reform*, Aurora, Garamond Press.

Aronson, Jane & Sheila Neysmith (1999). "The Retreat of the State and Long-Term Care Provision: Implications for Frail Elderly People, Unpaid Family Carers and Paid Home-Care Workers," in Pat Armstrong and Pat Connelly (eds.), *Feminism, Political Economy and the State: Contested Terrain*, Toronto, Canadian Scholar's Press.

Assistant Deputy Minister (1999). Letter from the Assistant Deputy Minister of Health and Long-term Care to the Community Care Access Centres, July 23.

Browne, Paul Leduc (2000). *Unsafe Practices: Restructuring and Privatization in Ontario Health Care*, Ottawa, Canadian Centre for Policy Alternatives.

Denton, Margaret et al. (2000). "Healthy Work Environments in Home-Care Agencies," *Journal of Occupational Health and Safety*, 16:5, 419-427.

Denton, Margaret et al. (1999). "Work-Related Violence and the OHS of Home-Health-Care Workers," *Women's Voices in Health Promotion*, Toronto, Canadian Scholar's Press, 45-60.

Frketich, J. (2002). "Elderly care agency closing," *Hamilton Spectator*, A1.

Frketich, J. (2002). "VHA Homemakers join to say goodbye," *Hamilton Spectator*.

Haiven, Larry (1995). "Industrial Relations in Health Care: Regulation, Conflict and Transition to the 'Wellness Model'," in Gene Swimmer & M. Thompson (eds.), *Public Sector Collective Bargaining in Canada : Beginning of the End or End of the Beginning?* Kingston, Queen's University, Industrial Relations Centre, 236-271.

HDHC (2000). *Directions for Long Term Care Planning*, Hamilton, Hamilton District Health Council (www.hdhc.ca).

HRDC (2001). *Setting the Stage: What Shapes the Home Care Labour Market*, Ottawa, Canadian Home Care Resources Study (www.homecarestudy.ca/en/news/docs/highlights-final.pdf).

Huang, R. (2000). "Some homecare workers to lose job as strike ends," *The Globe and Mail*.

Korpi, Walter (1998). "Power Resources Approaches vs Action and Conflict: On Causal and Intentional Explanations in the Study of Power," in J. S. O'Connor and G. M. Olsen (eds.), *Power Resources Theory and the Welfare State: A Critical Approach*, Toronto, University of Toronto Press, 37-69.

Lukits, A. (2002). "Patronage games? Tories compile list for home care board: No place for partisanship in essential health services, Liberal critics charge," *Kingston Whig-Standard*.

OACCAC (2000). *Human Resources: A Looming Crisis in the Community Care System in Ontario*, Scarborough, Ontario Association of Community Care Access Centres, (www.oaccac.on.ca/papers/HR_Position_paper.pdf).

O'Connor, Denise (1999). "Long-Term Care Reform and Community Care Access Centres in Ontario: The Effectiveness of Managed Competition," Hamilton, unpublished manuscript.

OCSA (2000). *The Effect of Managed Competition on Home Care in Ontario: Emerging Issues and Recommendations*, Toronto, Ontario Community Support Association (www.ocsa.on.ca).

OHHCPA & OCSA (2001). *Building a High Performance Home and Community Support System in Ontario*, Toronto, Ontario Home Health Care Providers' Association & Ontario Community Support Association joint position paper (www.ocsa.on.ca).

Pal, Leslie (1997). *Beyond Policy Analysis*, Scarborough, Nelson.

RNAO, 1999. *Reclaiming a Vision: Making Long-term Care Community Services Work*, Toronto, Registered Nurses Association of Ontario (www.rnao.org).

Urquhart, Ian (2001). "Harris hints at changes to home care." *The Toronto Star*.

Zeytinoglu, Isik U. (2000). "A Critical Review of Flexible Labour: Gender, Race and Class Dimensions of Economic Restructuring," *Restructuring and Women's Work*, 27: 3-4, 97-120.

Notes

[1] I would like to thank my supervisor, Charlotte Yates, for her support and her comments on this and an earlier version of this paper. I would also like to thank Paul Leduc Browne and the two independent readers for their comments on an earlier version of this paper.

[2] The author attended the Walkerton Inquiry the day Mr. Harris testified.

[3] This is an estimate of what front-line agencies spend. It has been estimated that CCACs spend between 20 percent and 35 percent of their budget on their administrative structures. (OHHCPA & OCSA, 2001)

[4] The CCAC model is very expensive. For example, CCACs consume about 30 percent of home-care dollars in Hamilton. Of that 30 percent, 55 percent of expenditures go to case management, 23 percent to administration, and the balance to equipment and medical supplies (according to the Hamilton CCAC 2002 annual report). Case managers are the gatekeepers of the system, but provide no direct service. On the (conservative) assumption that service providers incur administrative costs of 15 percent and a profit margin of 5 percent, the proportion of the home-care budget going to direct service is about $0.56 on every dollar. That is without taking into account the costs incurred by the Ministry of Health and Long-Term Care.

5   From an employer handbook. The contracts between CCACs and agencies roll personal support work and homemaking services into one price, although the skill levels are specified when a case is assigned to a provider.

6   This was a change instituted by the Harris government. Previously the qualifications were different. This change marked the beginning of the retention crisis.

Chapter 5
Care, Power, and Commodification[1]
Paul Leduc Browne

Introduction

Home care's growing prominence and increasing receipt of government monies in Ontario have gone hand in hand with its subjection to processes of commercialization and rationalization, much like other parts of the health-care system. In recent years, these processes have mainly been institutionalized by way of managed competition. Not surprisingly, the latter has received growing attention from social researchers and policy analysts. This final chapter will argue that managed competition exacerbates the effects of power structures already embedded in the division of home care labour, intensifying the clash between values intrinsic to the care relationship and the very different values imported into the care process by bureaucratic rationalization and commodification.

Home care as it exists today is characterized by a variety of purposes defined by various agents: governments; not-for-profit and for-profit enterprises; waged and unwaged workers; users and their families. Their many respective purposes are neither identical, nor always in harmony. This is reflected not merely in their divergent priorities, but also in the various ways in which they define the very nature of care and the ways in which they approach it—as a public service, as a business, as a job, as a calling, as a partnership, as a 'friendship.' No single perspective represents the exclusive truth about home care. Instead, each is embedded in, and informs, a relationship to practice, a set of values, needs and interests, and as such represents *a* truth. Some 'truths,' however, are truer than others (in the sense that they are more encompassing and better reflect fundamental relationships)—and some are more powerful. There is no question that certain positions in the division of labour confer greater power not only to determine what will be done, but also how to think and talk about it. The dominant versions of the truth are not necessarily the most accurate or encompassing, unfortunately.

Canada's federal and provincial governments define home care as "An array of services which enables clients incapacitated in whole or in part to live at home, often with the effect of preventing, delaying or substituting for long-term care or acute care alternatives" (Federal/Provincial/Territorial Working Group on Home Care, 1990). Defining care as an array of services presents considerable advantages. Formal care is a large-scale public enterprise involving the expenditure of some $2 billion of public money in Ontario today, as well as the mobilization of thousands of workers. It is mandated by law and regulated by the state. It is purchased and sold on the market like any other commodity. To define it as a *service*, rather than *care*, gets us away from sentimental ideas of it as a 'labour of love,' akin to care in the family, from the conflation of 'caring for' and 'caring about' (Neysmith, Baines, Evans, 1998; Leira, 1994), ideas which have been part and parcel of the subordination of women in society. It has more in common with other commercial or public services than with relations among kin.

Such definitions embody the government's 'truth' about home care. However, they do not encompass the full reality of carework, both waged and unwaged. The pressures arising from the introduction of managed competition in Ontario home care have highlighted divisions, which shall be spelled out here, between public authorities, private and non-profit agencies, waged and unwaged care workers, and care users. Yet, such tensions are at the very least latent in any situation in which the ability to care (i.e. the labour power of caregivers) is a commodity, in which the general interest is defined in abstraction from the immediate interests of care workers and users, indeed in which the division of labour translates into divisions of class, gender, and "race." I shall argue here that care is a complex whole with many different facets. The division of labour between public, non-profit and for-profit agencies, as well as between waged and unwaged caregivers, conceals this unity, making it rather appear to us as a sum of discrete services. Which aspects of care have the greatest visibility, and which disappear from view (as well as from official recognition, public funding, and the allocation of work time), is in no small part determined by who has the political and economic power to set the home care agenda, i.e. who has the power to determine the goals of the home care labour process. A key issue in this respect is how to reconcile the interests of care users, care workers, and the general public within the overall framework of publicly financed programs.

Care as a Labour Process

Caregiving is intellectually, emotionally, and physically demanding labour. "Caregiving involves several sets of skills and norms and requires the integration of menial, mental, and emotional skills [...] the combination of 'hand, brain, and heart' grounded in the dependent other's lack of capability to care for herself or himself is the salient feature of the caring process." (Leira, 1994:189.) Ideally, it works on bodies and emotions to produce and enhance social relationships not just of well-being, but of 'better-being' (mieux-être).

Carework comprises many different tasks, which have become the respective provinces of an array of waged and unwaged caregivers: registered nurses, physiotherapists, occupational therapists, speech-language therapists, personal support workers, companions, etc. (See Table 1). For all the diversity brought about by the division of labour, home care is first and foremost bodywork (Twigg, 2000a, 2000b). The material that caregivers labour upon is the human body—and furthermore the human body laid waste by age and illness. Those who care for the sick and elderly do not perform antiseptic, sanitized services. Many regularly work with excrement, and other bodily fluids and wastes. Caregivers work close to the limit of what society allows itself to accept or articulate—dirt, sexuality, illness, death.

This material labour is necessarily conjoined with emotional labour. The caregiver labours upon the body of the care recipient, while "managing feeling and using self to ensure that others (customers and clients) feel good and cared for."[2] (Aronson & Neysmith, 1996) Emotional labour involves considerable professionalism and skill.[3] As Nicky James puts it: "When emotions are thought to be 'irrational' it is hard to associate them with organization, yet managing them requires anticipation, planning, time-tabling and trouble-shooting as does other 'work,' paid and unpaid."(James, 1989, 27)

As the following quotation makes clear, the specific character of this emotional labour is embedded in unique personal relationships as a result of taking place in the home:

Home health care is an incredibly personal service, more so than hospital-based health care (...). You go into a hospital and you not only have no choice as to who is going to care for you, you don't expect choice, and you are out of your element, out of your environment, you are in a place where you don't expect to have any control. [...] When you go into somebody's home (and I've been on that end of it too), being the person going into the person's home, that's their environment, they are used to controlling their own environment and the hair in the back of their neck goes up when somebody else thinks they can exert that control. In any case, because you can control it—and it's one of the few things you can control—you demand that. In order to get around that, professionals and lay people going into people's homes learn to work within that environment, learn to garner your friendship in order to exert their professional influence, they learn how to become your friend, because you are more likely to accept a change from a friend than you are from a power source. We in home health care, speaking of the front-line level, we learned to work that culture, to meet our needs as professionals to do

Table 1

Community support services	Homemaking services	Personal support services	Professional services
Meal services Transportation Caregiver support services Adult day programs Home maintenance and repair Friendly visiting Security checks or reassurance services Social or recreational services Equipment, supplies and other goods	Housecleaning Laundry, ironing, mending Shopping, banking, paying bills Planning menus, preparing meals Caring for children Equipment and supplies	Personal hygiene activities Routine personal activities of living Equipment, supplies or other goods	Nursing Occupational therapy Physiotherapy Social work Speech-language pathology Dietetics Equipment, supplies or other goods

Source: *Statutes of Ontario, 1994*, Chapter 26 (*Long-Term Care Act, 1994*), s. 2 (3-7).)

our work, very differently than we learn to do it in the hospitals. It's one of the major practice differences, how you exert that control. When I was a 19-year-old new graduate nurse working at a floor in a hospital, I could easily walk into the room of a person I had never seen and say, "Hello, take off your clothes, put on that ugly blue gown, I want you to pee in this little thing and I want you to do this, do this, do this." And you do it. If I tried to do that in somebody's home, forget it! They'll say, "By the way, you are not coming in right now, because I am having my neighbour over for tea, so you are coming in later. I don't find it easy to get in and out of blue gowns, I have worn over-the-head gowns my entire life and I am wearing one now, and that's the way it's going to be. [...] The College of Nurses requires you to maintain this client-nurse relationship, but you can do that in such a way that the client really thinks you are a friend, but you are a nurse. But they don't see it that way." (Interview with CCAC executive, February 2001)

As these comments illustrate, the emotional labour of caring involves techniques designed to manage the relationship and expedite the tasks to be accomplished.

However, it would be mistake to treat the relationship as one of mere manipulation of the 'client' by the nurse. As the quotation indicates, the person who receives care is not a lump of clay manipulated by the caregiver, but an active participant in the labour process: "production and consumption occur in parallel, and users and workers are co-producers of care." (Twigg, 2000a, 121) To be sure, home care is mostly spoken of as a service provided by a professional to a client, customer or patient. (Increasingly, home care in Ontario substitutes for hospital-based acute care [see Daly in this volume], although it should not be reduced to this. In fact, most home care is carried out by unwaged caregivers.) But although we speak of caregivers and care recipients, carework is in fact mostly a joint effort, a collaboration between the two. As Twigg adds: "It is in the dynamics of the care encounter that the nature of what is produced is defined; production and consumption collapse into one another."[4]

Caregiving cannot be anonymous. It always involves the formation of a *personal*, physical and emotional relationship.[5] One does not wipe someone's bottom the way one would swipe the bar code on a tin of soup at the supermarket check-out counter. This may seem crude and self-evident, yet it is important to bear it in mind in an age when many labour processes have been or are becoming automated, or are performed in an impersonal, standardized manner, as we shall see presently.[6]

> Above all the close interpersonal nature of bodycare means that the principles of efficiency and of care are in conflict to a significant degree. Efficiency suggests that production should follow the model of MacDonald's with an emphasis on repeatability, on efficiencies of scale, on standardized interactions and limited involvement, but "care" is structured differently. Care requires that the response be highly individual, specific to that person and to that moment. It is by its very nature interactive, forged at the front line and cannot be separated from that setting or that interaction. Its remit is also unbounded, resting as it does on a response to the needs of the person as a whole rather than specific and localized care deficits. Care rests on an unbounded ethic that is in conflict with the focused, instrumental nature of waged work (...). (Twigg, 2000a, 122)

Beyond the tasks to be carried out (the IV, the bath, help in dressing, physiotherapy), the specific, personal relation of care production is both its foundation and its product. For those in need of care, the relationship with the caregiver is the foundation of trust and security—or their opposite. It is also, for many elderly people bound to their homes, the only immediate human contact with the "outside." In holding disease, decay and death at bay, a good care relationship also maintains and strengthens the care recipient's sense of self, dignity, and autonomy. For the care worker, the creation of such relationships is also a crucial source of meaning and fulfilment in a job that is physically and emotionally very demanding, but pays very little money (although this characterization of course does not apply so much to nurses, who enjoy decent wages, high professional status, and considerable public esteem).[7] The material labour of care is necessarily a social practice that transforms those who accomplish it.

The waged caregiver is therefore a professional, yet also a friend of a certain kind (Saillant & Gagnon, 2000). Francine Saillant has quoted recipients of care as describing their caregivers as friends, but "not friends like their other friends."[8] The caregiver is a stranger, yet also very intimate. Such a relationship offers enormous potential for people in need and their families. The former often find it much easier to receive intimate care from a stranger than from kin.[9] The latter may be content to surrender some aspects of care to a stranger, rather than be confronted with taboo situations (e.g., a parent's nudity) or ones that require special skills.[10] (Professional carework, it should be stressed, does not supplant, but complements care offered by friends and family.)

The dialectic of distance and proximity is a tightrope that both caregiver and care recipient have to cross successfully together. Excessive proximity could involve loss of self for the caregiver—or domination of the care recipient. Being too distant could reduce the care recipient to the status of a passive object. It is a delicate dance, which requires tact and forbearance as much as generosity and intimacy on both sides. Caregivers must learn to establish limits—indeed, waged caregivers are trained to do so—both in order to protect themselves and to generate the greatest possible autonomy for those for whom they care.

In sum, care is at best a holistic process in which care givers and recipients jointly define needs and work to address them, creating a sustained relationship of trust. However, care does not take place in an ideal world. Care givers and recipients must navigate treacherous waters, steering clear *inter alia* of the reduction of the workers to the status of domestics (where giving becomes oppression), the workers' transformation into pseudo-relatives (where the worker's free act of giving is enmeshed in the logic of kinship structures[11]), or the reduction of care to a mere exchange value. Simultaneously, the care user must not be reduced to the mere object of a service, the material substratum of the caregivers' activity or the passive consumer of a commodity. Nor, however, must the users be regarded as so empowered that much of the work can be offloaded onto them and their families.

Finally, the social relations of class, 'race' and gender pervade care, as they do society as a whole (Twigg, 2000a; Neysmith & Aronson, 1997). There is no point in hoping that care could somehow remain impervious to the effects of such structures of power and oppression.

Retrenchment and the Rationing of Care

A good care relationship depends on several conditions: respect, freedom, time, trust, giving (Saillant & Gagnon, 2000, 154-157). In home care, vulnerable people receive strangers into their homes and come to depend upon them. While a *service* may be performed in an impersonal way, the emotional work of *care* in conditions of forced intimacy requires trust, i.e. the formation of a personal bond. *Time* is particularly essential in this respect. When it comes to care, the only 'quality time' is 'quantity time.' It takes time to dispel insecurity and to build confidence (Saillant & Gagnon, 2000, 107, 155-156).

Care requires time—time to perform the various forms of bodywork, time to manage emotions, time to build and cement relationships, in brief, time for dialogue. Such time is available at the high end of the private market, where customers can afford to pay high fees to purchase it. In general, however, time is too costly to be readily available to many people when they must pay for it privately. In the public sector, time has also grown excessively dear, as the overriding imperative of cost restraint has pervaded every ministry and every program. Although there are expenditures on supplies and equipment in home care (for figures see Browne, 2000), wages make up the bulk of the costs. Reducing the latter has therefore meant finding ways of economizing on the expenditure of labour power, i.e. reducing the time available to home care users. Commenting on the U.S. scene, Andrew Szasz writes:

> Theoretically, agencies could hold down labour costs either through labour *market* strategies—lowering the occupational

skill mix, holding down employee compensation, and increasing the use of part-time employment—or by changing the labour *process* to increase the amount of useful (i.e., compensable) work performed by employees. A combination of labour market conditions and restrictive federal regulations severely limited opportunities for cost savings through wage cuts or skill-mix changes. Targeting the labour process proved to be the only viable option... (Szasz, 1990, 199)

All of this happened in Ontario health care in the 1990s (Armstrong et al., 2000; Browne, 2000). In hospitals, wages were held down, nurses were increasingly hired on a part-time basis, unregulated workers replaced nurses in many cases. Some of this was accomplished by moving many tasks from the hospital to the home. In addition, the labour process was changed: invisible and "unproductive" emotional work was notably discouraged.

In home care, both the labour market strategies and labour process rationalization have been pursued. Provincial regulation of personal support workers' wages kept the latter low (on average $10-$12 per hour [OCSA, 1999; OHHCPA, 1999]), but still well above the dismal minimum wage. Faced with managed competition, employers sought to push down employees' compensation on other fronts, such as benefits, and expenses (Browne, 2000). Other strategies were implemented too: shift from full-time to part-time work, intensification of the work, skill-mix changes. *In particular, the average length of visits was cut down and more visits were packed into a day.* The work has also been speeded up. Workers were allotted shorter time spans for each home visit and were expected to make more visits per work day. Furthermore, the work became more complex and demanding at every level.

But the shift in home care from chronic care to acute-care substitution has involved other obvious changes, notably a significant *work transfer* (Glazer, 1993, 1988) from hospitals to the home, from nurses to unregulated workers, and from waged to unwaged workers (Browne, 2000). Nurses increasingly do in the home a range of tasks formerly done in hospital, as unregulated workers do the work that nurses formerly did, and as unwaged caregivers fill in the gaps left by the paid workforce. In some places, notably larger urban centres, registered nurses reported to me that they only look after acute-care patients. Such care is much more technical and specialized. The work they previously did, in particular with elderly, chronic care patients, is increasingly being done by unregulated personal support workers or by informal caregivers, whose time is also being squeezed. The result is the exacerbation of the omnipresent contradictions between formal care and substantive needs, between what can be provided from above and what is needed from below:

> Body time is different from the clock time of industrial production or of science. It cannot be measured out, cut, put together, abstracted in the way that clock time—and to some degree service-time—can be. The needs of the body cannot be saved up and dealt with once a week. This is time that stops and starts in an arbitrary way. The time of domestic crisis only starts ticking once the old person has slipped on the stairs. It is the disjunction between these forms of time and logic of service delivery rooted in clock time that causes many of the tensions in community care... (Twigg, 2000, 100-101)

In these conditions, the system is saved from the consequences of its own logic only by the intervention of waged and unwaged caregivers (both kin and volunteers), who give of their time and effort to stop the gaps and hold back the tide of morbidity and misery. As long as this continues, the "rational" institutions can persist in the pretense that they are doing a good job, pointing to quantitative performance indicators as proof of their efficiency.

> This model does not operate in practice as it appears to in managerial designs that leave out nurses and family members as active agents. The design is assessed in terms of an efficiency standard that values fewer days in hospital. All players recognize that many patients will need more care, and assume that it will be delivered at home by the family. In this private sphere, who will do the work, under what conditions,

and with what quality control is not the concern of a public institution. (Neysmith, 2000, 11)

The purpose of care ought to be the maximization of home-care recipients' freedom and autonomy. In a good care relation, the worker shows respect for the other by treating her as an active subject, not a passive object. This means encouraging and nurturing the care recipient's dignity and autonomy as much as possible, notably by creating the physical conditions in which such dignity can be maintained. Yet, as a result of expenditure restrictions, CCACs reluctantly cut back on the hours of care they delivered and ceased to provide home support services, such as housecleaning. (Independent, 2001; Record, 2001; Review, 2001; Star, 2001; Weekly, 2001; Whig Standard, 2001a, 2001b) Many people receiving care in their homes will be forced to live in more insalubrious, unhygienic or even dangerous environments, or to give up their homes entirely. This is conducive neither to dignity nor to autonomy. It also forces the workers to labour in unhealthy conditions (see Hollander and Tessaro, 2001, on the health impacts of forms of home support such as cleaning).

Commodification and Rationalization of Care

Managed competition has exacerbated skill-mix changes, downward pressures on wages, and the other trends just mentioned. But managed competition merely makes more difficult a situation in which the power to define needs, and to invest work, time and money, is not vested in workers and users in the home, but in governmental and quasi-governmental institutions that present themselves as the gatekeepers of public finances and the representatives of the public interest. The fundamental issue is the social division of labour, by virtue of which governments and their proxies, purportedly acting on behalf of society, define social needs, determine the means of satisfying them, and contract out the work of doing so to non-governmental agencies. The latter in turn hire caregivers to do the actual work. The entire process defines distinct relationships to work, and thus the class positions of workers, clients/consumers, employers, contractors, policymakers.

Public authorities contract out work, and firms in turn hire employees, to execute their purposes. They do not wish their contractors or workers to involve themselves in any other activities while on the job, and they wish the mandated tasks to be performed with maximum efficiency. While none would deliberately set out with the goal of harming the interests of home-care users, they are nevertheless driven by a variety of public policy and commercial goals, which do not per se coincide with those interests. In order to ensure both that their goals (and only their goals) are pursued and that their costs are kept at a minimum (Braverman, 1974), businesses and bureaucratic organizations rationalize their operations with a view to affording managers maximum oversight and control over the labour process. This is perfectly logical. The problem is the inherent heterogeneity of these purposes, of the full needs of the care users, and of the interests of the workers.

For an agency that sets policy and funds programs, the key issue is how to ensure that the organizations and individuals it employs to execute the work achieve the prescribed objectives in the most efficient way. From this vantage point, the time during which workers perform their tasks is a 'black box' that must be made to conform to the invested inputs and desired outputs. A typical way to gain control of care and guarantee "value for money" is to break open the "black box" by defining care in terms of measurable factors. These indicators can then be used to make workers and consumers "accountable."

For persons actually carrying out the work or receiving care in the home, the big question mark is instead the policy goals defined elsewhere. Do they truly correspond to the needs caregivers and care recipients experience, and how does the policy process either facilitate or impede fulfilment of those needs?

The first perspective, typically mediated by quantitative indicators, regards quality as an issue of accountability—is the mandate being implemented? Are the *services* that have been purchased being delivered? Is the purchaser getting value for money? From the second perspective, quality appears as the immediacy of *care* needs and working conditions.[12]

The first perspective is at the heart of much critical debate and analysis today. It drives a considerable, multi-pronged campaign to design and implement ways of evaluating care. *It is evident that this issue only arises because of the division of labour and resources within the home-care system, where those who pay are not the same as those who decide what should be done, who are not the same as those who carry out the work, who in turn are not the same as those whose needs are ultimately supposed to be the* raison d'être *of the whole process.* In the light of this division of labour, it is possible to see that the labour process does not look the same from the standpoint of the political and bureaucratic authorities that formulate the system's policy goals, as it does from the standpoint of caregivers and care recipients in the home. Indeed, in an era of cost restraint and privatization, these perspectives are in fact likely to be in contradiction and conflict with each other.

Faced with budget cuts and, in the case of for-profit institutions and agencies, the imperative to turn a profit, managers throughout the health-care system have restructured and rationalized their production processes and labour forces. The quantitative analysis of work (e.g., time and motion studies) has been a key tool in the rationalization of labour, enabling managers to break down and redesign the labour process so as better to control it.[13] Adam Smith long ago showed how the production of commodities such as pins could be speeded up and made much more efficient by breaking the process down and having workers perform only specific operations. Under such conditions, a worker may accomplish the prescribed task with greater skill and speed, increasing productivity. It matters little in such a context whether the task consists in making pinheads or jabbing needles in a person's arm in order to gather blood samples. Smith demonstrated that businesses could realize increased profits by breaking down the labour process into its component parts and assigning as much of the work as possible to employees who could be paid the lowest wages. (Smith, 1776) This is a general trend throughout society (Braverman, 1974; Burawoy, 1999, 1985; Foster, 1999), as well as in the health care system. (Armstrong, 2001; Armstrong et al., 2000, 1997, 1994; Armstrong & Armstrong, 1996; White, 1990)

The rationalization of the labour process highlights some aspects of labour and conceals others, defines some as meaningful and worthwhile and others as irrelevant. Rationalization operates like a projector in a dark room. It makes certain objects visible and leaves the others in darkness. In the process, the activities most difficult to quantify, measure and control have tended to be marginalized.[14] The tendency here is for only the measurable parts of care to be recognized, while the relationship components remain "invisible and unnamed."[15] (Armstrong, 2001; Aronson & Neysmith, 1996) Certain features of labour, typically the most quantifiable ones, get retained and highlighted as most conducive to these goals, while other aspects of the work are purged. Managerial rationalization in a sense places workers' labour on a Procrustean bed, amplifying and extending some activities, while cutting out others. To quote Sheila Neysmith:

> As resources become scarce, visible work is given priority. For example, caring labour is reduced to counting the number of meals delivered, baths given, sheets changed, etc. The emotional and mental work that underpins the tasks is slotted as time allows but not considered essential. Ironically, although women may be hired for these jobs because of their skills in dealing with people's feelings, they are given no credit for these skills. (Neysmith, 1998, 237)

Rather than being regarded as a complex totality of physical and emotional labour[16], care comes to be regarded as a set of discrete measurable tasks[17], which can then be reduced in number to save time.[18]

At the present time, managerial technologies are targeting nursing practice more directly than patient classification did, putting individual caregivers' decisions about their practice more securely within the managerial sphere of influence. "Clinical pathways," for instance, is one current form of planning that some hospitals have implemented to streamline treatment, including nursing care, and to expedite patients' movements through costly hospital stays. Expediting a patient's movement by having staff adhere to a plan such as a clinical pathway means that the nurse caring for the patient will eliminate all but essential care in order to meet the plan's targets. Not doing so could result in a variance that requires explanation, a form of text-mediated enforcement of the protocol in nurses' practice. The literature is now using the term "non-value added" to refer to those activities that nurses would be expected to drop to meet targets. Managers attempting to achieve their organization's new efficiency and effectiveness goals are looking for ways to identify and reduce nurses' non-value-added work in order to reduce the number of nurses needed to care for patients. (Campbell, 2000, 190)

Rationalizing carework is a problematic endeavour, however, for *care* is not just any kind of service, nor does it just deliver specific goods or products. For example, it does not just consist in giving someone a bath or physiotherapy; it is crucially a particular way of bathing that person. Its definition as a sum of services (for example in Figure 1) does not reflect its rich complexity. Indeed, it could be argued that it breaks down a holistic, complex process into a sum of discrete things.

This is not merely a question of semantics, nor is it accidental. It reflects the clash between bureaucratic and commercial imperatives on the one hand, and the intrinsic relationship between caregiver and user on the other. The definition of home care as a collection of *discrete services* is more than a convenient description compiled for the sake of information. These are items purchased by CCACs. There is no question that the buying and selling of carework on the market is greatly facilitated if it can be reduced to discrete measurable activities that can be priced in a standardized fashion.[19] Managed competition drives the consolidation of this process. From a commercial or bureaucratic perspective, reducing care to a sum of services thus has the advantage of turning an unbounded process into something that can be quantified, measured and *priced*. The qualitative and holistic aspects of care do not lend themselves to this. It is ironic that the word "care" only appears once in the definition quoted from the Long-term

Care Act at the beginning of the chapter—and then it does not refer to the person receiving the "service," but to care for that person's children!

The paradigm of measurement is also essential to current efforts at cost containment in the public sector. In the name of "accountability," it has been found desirable to define the labour paid for with tax dollars in measurable terms. The introduction of "businesslike" practices is a key feature of the new public management. (Browne, 2000; Shields & Evans, 1998) In the home care field, this became especially true with the creation of the community care access centres as non-profit organizations fully funded by the provincial government and answerable to it for their expenditure of public monies. When the CCACs engage in quality control, they attempt to measure the performance of these discrete activities.[20]

The drive to make care *measurable* is thus driven by a number of related factors, notably a bureaucratic will to control and a neo-liberal will to commercialize. As discussions surrounding international trade and investment negotiations have shown, the itemization of specific services is a crucial aspect in opening up whole sectors of socio-economic activity to international commercial competition. (Sanger, 2001; Sinclair, 2000; Shrybman, 1999) Feminist scholarship has also shown the gender bias of the paradigm of measurement. (Armstrong, 2001)

Home care is even more of a "black box" than other health care institutions, because it takes place in a "private" residence, away from the scrutiny of managers. Unlike hospitals, the production of care in the home takes place in a "hidden," private territory not subject to external control to the same degree. (Twigg, 2000a, 121) This makes it hard for organizations to control the production process. Managers establish practice guidelines and quality standards, and then rely on reporting protocols, surveys and other measures to try to check on their implementation. The introduction of telehomecare promises to change this radically, since it will offer managers unprecedented opportunities to supervise and control the labour process of their workers.

Despite the rationalization of their labour process, good caregivers constantly try to provide little "extras." (Saillant & Gagnon, 2000) To cite the title of a fine article on this subject: "You're not just in there to do the work!" (Neysmith and Aronson, 1996)

> One of the classic features of this tension is the existence of "extras": work undertaken by staff outside the official schedule of duties. "Extras" are a recurring feature of home care, and one found across welfare systems. Typically, they cover things like: taking the client Christmas shopping, making birthday cakes, running round with a plate of Sunday dinner, buying underwear, taking the cat to the vet, bringing a husband round to clear the gutters, popping back in the evening to tuck the person in; and all of these featured in the interviews. Some extras represent things not provided by the welfare system but that are needed or valued by the client; others represent the shortfall between what the system is willing to allocate and what the worker feels is needed. Either way, extras are unrecompensed labour. (Twigg, 2000a, 170)

As long as it does not conflict with "official" duties and is not unsafe, managers will often tolerate such activity, while praising the human qualities and dedication of the caregivers. In any truly holistic concept of care, the "extras" would be recognized as an integral part of the work and would be integrated into the overall work plan, not left to the whim and generosity of the individual worker. But because the rationalization of the labour process has split it asunder, reducing formal care to a set of rationalized, costed services, much of care becomes invisible or becomes identified as something peculiar to the workers who do it.

> Managers have always been aware of these activities, and in large degree have turned a blind eye. Indeed many, in praising the home care workforce for their dedication and commitment, cite their involvement in extras. This is not seen primarily as an aspect of the work, so much as a result of a personal feature of the workers—their caring and kindly natures. That character is praised—sometimes to the skies—but not rewarded financially. It is regarded as something that arises naturally from their character as caring women. It is

not what they *do* but who they *are*. Extras thus represent work that is extracted on the basis of the traditional gender contract, but not officially recognized or recompensed in the formal one. (Twigg, 171-172)

From the point of view of the rationalization of care, the "informal" care that caregivers fit in to the interstices of their formal tasks thus appears as an "irrational residue" in the labour process, the rationalization of which is being driven by government retrenchment and managed competition.[21]

Of course, were we to grasp carework holistically, we would see nothing "irrational" in such gifts. On the contrary, we should regard them as flowing logically from the very holistic nature of the care relationship. For *care*giving is also care*giving*. Even when it is done by waged workers, it is always more than a mere service performed for money.

In the light of patriarchal and paternalistic ideologies both of women's work and of charity, such a statement needs to be qualified. As Julia Twigg points out, when the "extra" work is neither formally recognized nor remunerated, it is extracted from the workers "on the basis of the traditional gender contract." Yet, giving need not consist only of sublime martyrdom or maternal self-sacrifice. It could also represent a bond of reciprocity and solidarity, the creation of a mutual indebtedness that sustains an ongoing, even deepening relationship. This would also differ from the marketplace, where people seek to obtain what they need from others without becoming personally involved with them. The market exchange of goods and services is (theoretically) based on a principle of exact equivalence. Where there is debt, everyone's goal is to liquidate it as quickly as possible—thus ending the basis of the relation to the other. (Godbout, 2000, 151-152) In a gift relationship, by contrast, the point is to perpetuate the bond with the other.

The essential gift a caregiver can provide is time, time to look after physical needs, to talk, especially to listen—time to build a relationship. As Saillant and Gagnon (2000, 155) point out: "Time is a gift of self, even when it is remunerated; it blazes the path of reflexivity (between care givers and recipients and each for her/himself) and of the space to be taken." Clearly, the continuity of care is absolutely essential to its quality. Every time a new caregiver takes over, a new relationship must be forged. The special needs and habits of the care recipient need to be explained once again and, more importantly, trust must be established anew.[22]

It is interesting that we often try to give a little more than is required, in order to make our gifts appear more authentic, more genuine, more than the perfunctory fulfilment of a social duty. Similarly, to appear really good, care must always transcend the bounds of what is required or expected. At the same time, it must be limited so that the workers do not lose themselves. They must measure their time (though not in an accounting sense) to avoid burning out.[23] The crucial continuity of the relationship depends on their ability to sustain their gift of self over the long run. (Saillant & Gagnon, 2000, 155-156) However, in a system where labour power is a commodity measured in units of time, workers can only provide the necessary time at their own expense.

The workers are caught here in the contradiction between a bureaucratic mandate (translated into commercial contracts) to perform specific tasks in the allotted time and the holistic nature of care, reinforced both by an ethic of solidarity with the people to be cared for and by public perceptions of carework as a labour of love, i.e. something unlimited and selfless. Bound by contracts with the community care access centres, home care agencies require their employees to make a given number of visits per day and to carry out prescribed activities in each one. At the same time, the needs to be met are far deeper and more numerous, while the workers are motivated by solidarity, compassion and a sense of duty to do more than their mandate in order to meet those needs. Yet it becomes increasingly difficult for caregivers to reconcile the contradictory pressures, as constraints on their time and the specialization of their work force them to perform only the tasks allotted by their employers.

The aspects of the work that have been pushed aside by rationalization do not just disappear then, but keep cropping up.[24] In terms of the performance of the contracted tasks (operating dialysis machines, inserting IVs, bathing and dressing "clients"), they are like weeds in a garden, irrational residues in a rationalized environment. But attempts to stamp out these residues may have the same unintended consequences as industrial disregard for ecological sustainability. The "irrational" aspects may be essential to the cohesion of the labour process and their removal may result in its disintegration. To quote Sheila Neysmith again:

It may not seem like news that the system mediation work done by nurses is not specified as a nursing task and thus is lost in the reorganizing, but this has serious implications for patient-centred care—the title of the restructuring scheme. If nursing continues to be conceptualized and resourced as a set of tasks (...), when the current generation of nurses who hold things together with their unrecognized labour retire, dangerous gaps will appear in patient-centred care. (Neysmith, 2000, 11)

To be sure, many of the managers and executives of the agencies that provide home care are themselves nurses, as are the case managers in the community care access centres. The fault line between the 'care' and 'service' perspectives runs through their ranks and their practice.[25]

For example, the executive director of one non-profit agency that provides home care told me the following story:

I have a very good friend whose mother is in [a town in Ontario] (...) I've been there a couple of times when her home-care worker comes in the morning. She has cancer and she has home support weekly and the lady would come in. And when she found out who I was, she was very, very nervous that, somehow, I was going to report her. My friend's mother sleeps on the couch ever since her husband passed away— there's no way that she's going to sleep in the bedroom, so she sleeps on the couch—and this lady will come in (she's got a key to come in) while D. is sleeping and she will just sit quietly in the chair. Then she will put the kettle on and make a pot of tea and she will wait for D. to wake up. And then they have this pot of tea together and if D. wants a bath, then she baths her, you know, and does the tidying up, but mainly what she does—she recognizes what she's doing, I recognize what's she doing and so does D.—she is providing companionship for her and, you know, that's what [D.] wants. [Her care worker] makes sure that the house is tidy. But she is doing a very important function, you know, but when she found out I was with [the agency I am with], it took a lot to reassure her that if I knew that all my home support workers were acting the same way, I would be quite happy. [Interview with the author, December 2000]

Conversely, the director of another non-profit home-care agency told me that nurses no longer have time for such conversation and companionship. In response to my questions, she remarked that nurses might not be the individuals best suited to that role in any case, further suggesting that this function could be accomplished by bringing senior citizens together regularly in congregated settings, possibly while they receive specialized care. [Interview with the author, September 1999]

In a draft of an earlier study, I quoted the words of the director of a home-care agency, who had told me that nurses' work has changed and that they "no longer go in and have a cup of tea with the client." Representatives of a health-care lobby group criticized me harshly for quoting this, claiming that I was demeaning skilled professionals by suggesting that their difficult job had ever consisted in taking tea with the clients. Quite apart from the fact that the words were not mine, this reaction is interesting for what it says about the ideology of professionalism and the atomization of care. The implication is that spending some minutes speaking with the client over a cup of tea somehow means not working, shirking one's duty, or being unprofessional.

Yet, it should not require a great deal of anthropological insight to understand that "having a cup of tea" means performing a social ritual which inaugurates and cements a relationship between the caregiver and the care recipient. Of course, performance of such rituals requires time—the essential element of a good care relationship. But time is no longer available, as workers are rushed off their feet, dashing from one client to the next to accomplish the "real work" recognized by government funders.[26]

The status of carework in Ontario society today is such that it remains largely invisible as long as it is accomplishing its mission. It is only when it fails or is in some way lacking that it comes to be seen, and then negatively.[27] As Sheila Neysmith puts it: "Like prevention, the product is invisible; it exists in the negative form of distress rather than in the positive form of adjustment." (Neysmith, 1998, 237) Julia Twigg (2000a) points out that there is a continuity between care for the frail elderly and other forms of gendered activities, such as housework or child care. All involve a process of knitting, repairing or maintaining a reality in constant flux. Because of this sense of the work never being done and always needing to be taken up anew, carework seems unbounded and its temporality fluid. Although home care contracts may define care as a set of well-defined services to be performed at set times, in practice the needs to be met are often broader and the time needed to fulfil them always greater.[28]

This process is reinforced by the nature of the work, as well as by the way it has been gendered and racialized. Many of the difficult and unpleasant aspects of home care (e.g., dirt) are elided in public discourse. But that which is "invisible" in care (emotional labour, but also the work of tending to the bodies of others) has traditionally been identified as "women's work" and, as such, as "natural." Indeed, it has been regarded as so natural that it is not really regarded as work at all and certainly not as something that one would put a price on.[29]

Care is devalued because it is "women's work" and because its subject matter is quite literally "shit." (Twigg, 2000b) Those aspects of care which require some specialized knowledge and technical skills have been abstracted and made the preserve of professionals. The rest has been relegated to poorly paid, unregulated workers. These devalued parts of carework are very poorly remunerated and are disproportionately assigned to women of colour, often immigrants. There is a tendency among some professionals, who have been engaged in a decades-long struggle for increasing status, recognition and autonomy, to dissociate themselves from these subaltern tasks.

Other Aspects of the Loss of Continuity

Time is not only fleeting because CCACs provide fewer hours of care per month, or because more tasks are crammed into the hours remaining. It is also truncated when, by losing contracts in the tendering process, agencies disappear from communities in which they have been active for decades and are replaced by brand new companies. The inevitable turnover in personal support workers disrupts long-established relationships, patterns of work, and networks of trust (Browne, 2000), this despite the fact that continuity is widely recognized as one of the crucial principles of care.[30] Although community care access centres and the agencies to which they award contracts believe in retaining the workforce already in place, this has proven increasingly problematic in practice. Some workers do move from the losing to the winning agencies, but many do not, preferring to find employment in other health sectors (hospitals, nursing homes), communities, or even countries (see O'Connor in this volume).[31]

Managed competition further dislocates the labour process by the way it pits agencies against each other. Previously, even when different aspects of the work were done by different agencies, the latter used to meet regularly to exchange information and knowledge, and to coordinate their work. The bidding war put an end to this, compelling the non-profit organizations as much as the for-profit companies to conceal vital information about their finances, practices and workforce in order not to give away trade secrets and yield any market advantage to their competitors.

Given the size of their caseloads, CCAC case managers cannot have a detailed, hands-on knowledge of each person assigned to them, even though they are the only workers charged with a holistic knowledge of the care recipient. They rarely meet most of the people in their caseload face to face. Instead, they rely on input from the relatives, personal support workers, nurses, therapists, or physicians. Such input consists to a very great extent in brief voice-mail messages. Meanwhile, each of those providing it often has only an incomplete knowledge of the care recipient. Even within agencies, nurses and personal support workers spend far more time on the road, coming to the office much less frequently, even more sporadically.[32] There is not the same integration of experience and generation of collective knowledge as in the past, when care conferences involving all the providers were more regular and frequent.

Policy Directions

The division within the labour process between those who define the purposes of the work, those who actually do it, and those who appropriate its products, is not a new phenomenon. In an era when home care was much less prominent and money was more plentiful, governments left it to local public health departments, non-profit institutions and health-care professionals to determine and provide the appropriate forms of care. In a sense, home care goals were determined at different levels. Governments recognized need and formulated very general purposes; health-care professionals (including those managing local agencies) defined concrete care goals.

Public sector retrenchment and commercialization have changed all this. In the new era of accountability and total quality management, autonomy at every level of the system has been constrained by authorities at higher levels seeking greater control. More specific, detailed goals have been formulated at higher levels and imposed on the lower instances through legislation, regulation, policy, budgets, and accounting procedures. Interviews with their managers indicate that this has compelled many local provider agencies to run their operations in leaner, tighter fashion. As the overriding imperative has shifted from the provision of care to the cost-efficient—and, in the context of managed competition, profitable—delivery of services, significant changes have been made in home-care work: work transfer, speeding up, rationing, loss of continuity. The government and its agents may be able to point to a rising volume of nursing visits and homemaking hours. Quite apart from the fact that its funding cuts have compelled CCACs to reduce the hours of care they purchase per client, it is not clear that the government can also point to an increased quality of life for care workers and users, and an improved quality of relationships established between them. Certainly, these are concerns within the agencies that provide home-care services. There, the increasingly difficult working conditions and the worsening shortage of workers are constant and deepening preoccupations and sources of frustration. In our interviews with non-profit agencies, this concern a number of times even translated into doubt as to whether it was even worth continuing to work in the sector.

A number of steps must be taken immediately to address these issues. The Ontario government must follow through with the logic of the turn to community care which it and its predecessors have set in motion, and provide full and adequate funding to the long-term community care system. It must invest in training and hiring nurses, support workers and therapists, as well as increasing wages and benefits in the sector. Community Care Access Centres must be given the means to increase the care hours provided to their clients, as well as restore services they have cut, such as cleaning and food preparation, that play an important role in enabling people to stay at home and maintain their health. Much greater integration is needed between the hospitals, long-term care centres, home care and social services.

Beyond such vital measures, however, it will also be important to address the issue of power within carework, in order to ensure that the needs and interests of both workers and users are fully met. This means challenging the division of labour in which some define the goals and control the resources, others do the work, and others still are reduced to passive recipients of limited services.

What policy and program design changes could empower workers and users?

One option would seek to eliminate the conditions in which external authorities intervene in the individual care relation. This could take two forms.

1. The first would be the move to a "pure," unmediated, one-on-one relation between volunteer/family member and care recipient, in other words the abandonment of formal home care entirely. This is a complete non-starter. It simply negates the overwhelming need for any formal home care, throwing all the responsibility on users to find their own support and on informal caregivers to find the time and

resources to do the work. This option is impractical and unfair both to users and informal caregivers. It imposes an unconscionable and unrealistic burden on the latter in a social context in which most are already burdened with wage labour and caregiving duties, and in which the lion's share of the latter are borne by women. It is also unreasonable and inequitable to expect that all those in need of care will have access to family, friends or volunteers to care for them. Moreover, this option denies care users the contribution of professional caregivers— *l'étranger chez soi* (Saillant & Gagnon, 2000)—in the form of expertise, but also a certain distance, which is not available with kin and friends.

2. The demand for expertise and "distance" can be met through the direct purchase of care by the care recipient. This option is favoured by advocates of market solutions, because it is held to empower consumers to choose the nature, quality and price of their own services. Individuals purchase services directly and are their own case managers.

This option without question has attractive features for some users. As a consumer, the user has the freedom to choose between the services and providers available, and to select the most appropriate one. Furthermore, the user can also choose to change providers should the one selected prove inappropriate, inadequate, incompetent, or incompatible. This power to initiate and terminate the care relationship can give the user the sense of being much more in control of the care relationship.

Such a system would raise many questions about employment standards and conditions. As Carpenter points out:

> From the workers' point of view, there is a danger that such schemes will lead to a deterioration of pay and conditions, fragmentation of career structures and opportunities, and subordination to the whim of users. By rightly focusing singlemindedly on the human rights of users, there is nevertheless the danger of overlooking those of employed workers. In other words, there are conflicts of ideology and interest,

and a dialogue is only possible on the basis of recognizing and accepting that they exist. (Carpenter, 1994, 138-139)

From the user's standpoint, as is often the case in the marketplace, consumer freedom may in any case prove illusory. To begin with, one needs to have money in order to be a consumer. Many of the frail elderly live in poverty on modest incomes. To be sure, the government could distribute vouchers. That in turn raises two further questions: who would be entitled to the vouchers? And could such a system provide users with enough money, without greatly increasing government expenditures? On the issue of entitlement, there is a very big difference between a system which offers vouchers only on a means-tested, welfarist basis, and a universal system which makes them available to all. In the former case, one would end up with a kind of multi-tier, patchwork setup such as prevails in child care in Ontario.

But if entitlement were universal, could the government afford it? Economics suggests that prices will rise if a few suppliers deal with a multitude of small purchasers, rather than with one single purchaser, as is the case when the community care access centre brokers community care in a given geographical area. And if prices rose, would government be willing to match them in its home-care vouchers, or would the latter more likely stagnate, swiftly ceasing to cover the real cost of care, and thus restoring inequality in access to care? Conversely, if purchasers bypass the big agencies and hire individual caregivers directly, the opposite may occur: wages and working conditions may drop, and much of the work may be done on the black market.

But even were such objections to be met in a convincing way, there are other arguments against an individual-purchaser model. Care management represents a considerable range and quantity of work— collecting information about the services available on the market, investigating agencies, establishing the most appropriate mix of services, negotiating contracts, scheduling service delivery, monitoring quality, making payments, etc. Although some individuals may successfully recruit the best care for themselves, "empowering" individuals and families to be their own care managers would in general merely increase the burden of unwaged labour that women must perform, as

Sheila Neysmith has pointed out. The proposal also ignores the degree of expertise involved in care management: "Information and contacts are a form of knowledge and a source of power that professionals have and families do not. A family carer may be able to modify what is available, but it is truly a professional skill to advocate and manoeuvre in a complex system of health and social services." (Neysmith, 1998, 241)

3. This is not to deny the very real knowledge and energy of many service users (and/or their kin). It rather implies the need for brokers and advocates, and, at that, of a single broker, rather than many of them, in order to control costs. Managed competition in Ontario purports to address these issues by blending the market virtues of provider competition and consumer choice with the advantages of brokerage, the practice of case management, and the monopsonistic power of a single purchaser.

Yet real difficulties remain, as the contributors to this book have argued, because users' choices under the system are very limited. They pay the price of competition in the loss of continuity, while workers pay the price of competition by seeing their working conditions eroded. Most CCACs offer "clients" no choice of provider agency. One exception is the Kingston, Frontenac, Lennox & Addington CCAC, which requires each person on the caseload to choose a provider agency from a list of the agencies that have successfully bid on a contract.

As this chapter has argued, despite the extraordinary amount of words spent on it, accountability remains a major problem—both from the managerial perspective and from the standpoint of the service users. Accountability is limited, because case managers cannot assess the quality of the services they order except in partial and abstract ways. On the one hand, they conduct occasional visits with the clients and survey them using customer satisfaction questionnaires. But many vulnerable elderly service users may be reluctant to speak out openly about poor care (on the potential and limits of evaluation, see Williams et al., 2001). On the other hand, CCACs rely on a trail of written forms and voice-mail messages to determine that the services ordered have been delivered. But this trail tells them nothing about the actual quality of the care relationship, although it is undoubtedly useful from an administrative and cost-containment point of view.

There are intrinsic contradictions in the case managers' role. Their mandate is to guard the public purse and to be advocates for their "clients." When cost containment, cuts and rationing are the order of the day, these two priorities may be difficult, even impossible to reconcile. Case managers must also coordinate a "client's" care. This involves working closely with the provider agencies. Case managers may deal with managers and professionals of nursing homes, retirement homes, and home-care agencies over a number of years. Often, case managers have been recruited from the ranks of those organizations. In their work, they have much more frequent contact with those managers and professionals than with their "clients." The need to remain on good terms and build smooth working relationships may, at the very least, constrain or colour the ways in which case managers advocate for "clients" and the extent to which they do so. In extreme cases, there is the risk of cronyism.

The CCAC model reproduces divisions between individual and collectivity, "client" and "expert," and user and worker. Mick Carpenter's comments on British reforms applies also to Ontario:

1. [the managerial-consumerist model] is wholly individualist, deflecting attention away from the need also for collective empowerment, and from the influence of "race," gender and class inequalities on sickness and disability;

2. it sees care as a "product" to be delivered in pre-defined "packages" in ways that will encourage the expert role to be assumed, as before, if not by professionals then by managers, devaluing or ignoring the expertise of users—and also because the need to ration will require the repression of genuine user choice;

3. it perpetuates a divisive analytical distinction between consumer and producer, or user and worker that is not a satisfactory basis for a progressive community care which acknowledges the contribution of all participants to care. (Carpenter, 1994, 12)

Carpenter argues that we must rather develop a new understanding of the "active producers of care, with different types of expertise to contribute, whether as employed professionals or care staff, volunteers, informal carers, or the 'users' of services themselves." (Carpenter, 1994, 12) In opposition to individualistic and market-oriented approaches, this would imply working within the collective provision of care, to break down the institutional powers that weigh down on users and workers.

This implies a sharp challenge not only to caring for profit, but also to public administration, and a technocratic ideology of professionalism. The challenge is to invent models of policy-making, administration, and service delivery that transcend the impersonality, passivity and individualism bred by bureaucracy and the market. The work of care is collective: it brings caregivers and care recipients together in a joint labour process in the framework of public programs. It is a public good produced in the privacy of an individual's home. It places strangers in a relationship of great intimacy. In contrast with the impersonality of market and bureaucracy, the caring relationship addresses the care recipient's decreasing ability and diminishing autonomy in life, by creating a new personal bond through the gift of time and of self. Yet, unlike patriarchal relations of dependency, the relationship of care does not, ideally, institute the domination of worker over user or vice versa.

The tendency of both public- and private-sector bureaucracies is to drive ever further the rationalization and division of labour, increasing disparities and hierarchies, in order to cut costs and/or raise profits. The logic of care, by contrast, suggests the need for a holistic approach at odds with the fragmentation and quantification of the labour process. Just as the bureaucratic approach requires forms of accountability based on cost control, care as I have defined it implies a form of accountability based on the democratic association of workers, users and their families. This in turn cannot exist as an island of the blessed in the cold seas of a technocratic society, but calls for the integration of co-operative structures bringing together care, assistance with activities of daily living, transportation, housing, and nutrition.

Bibliography

Armstrong, Pat (2001). "Evidence-Based Health-Care Reform: Women's Issues," in Pat Armstrong, Hugh Armstrong & David Coburn (eds.), *Unhealthy Times. Political Economy Perspectives on Health and Care in Canada*, Toronto, Oxford University Press, 121-145.

Armstrong, Pat & Hugh Armstrong (1996). *Wasting Away: The Undermining of Canadian Health Care*, Toronto, Oxford University Press.

Armstrong, Pat, Hugh Armstrong, Ivy Bourgeault, Jacqueline Choinière, Eric Mykhalovsliy, Jerry P. White (2000). *"Heal Thyself." Managing Health Care Reform*, Toronto, Garamond Press.

Armstrong, Pat, Hugh Armstrong, Jacqueline Choinière, Eric Mykhalovsliy, Jerry P. White (1997). *Medical Alert*, Toronto, Garamond Press.

Armstrong, Pat, Hugh Armstrong, Jacqueline Choinière, Jerry P. White (1994). *Take Care, Warning Signals for Canada's Health Care*, with a foreword by Joel Lexchin, Toronto, Garamond.

Aronson, Jane & Sheila M. Neysmith (1996). "'You're Not Just in There to Do the Work': Depersonalizing Policies and the Exploitation of Home Care Workers' Labour," *Gender and Society*, 10:1, 59-77.

Braverman, Harry (1974). *Labor and Monopoly Capital. The Transformation of Work in the Twentieth Century*, New York, Monthly Review Press.

Browne, Paul Leduc (2000). *Unsafe Practices. Restructuring and Privatization in Ontario Health Care*, Ottawa, Canadian Centre for Policy Alternatives.

Browne, Paul (1992). "Reification and the Crisis of Socialism," in Jos. Roberts & Jesse Vorst (eds.), *Socialism in Crisis? Canadian Perspectives*, Halifax, Fernwood Books, 15-50.

Burawoy, Michael (1996). "A Classic of Its Time," *Contemporary Sociology*, 25: 3, May.

Burawoy, Michael (1985). *The Politics of Production. Factory Regimes Under Capitalism and Socialism*, London, Verso.

Campbell, Marie (2000). "Knowledge, Gendered Subjectivity, and the Restructuring of Health Care: The Case of the Disappearing Nurse," in Sheila Neysmith (ed.), *Restructuring Caring Labour: Discourse, State Practice, and Everyday Life*, Toronto, Oxford University Press, 2000.

Carpenter, Mick (1994). *Normality Is Hard Work: Trade Unions and the Politics of Community Care*, London, Lawrence & Wishart in association with Unison.

Federal/Provincial/Territorial Working Group on Home Care (1990). *Report on Home Care*, Ottawa, National Health and Welfare.

Foster, John Bellamy (1999). "A Classic of Our Time: *Labor and Monopoly Capital* After a Quarter-Century," *Monthly Review*, 50:8, January.

Gilain, Bruno, Marthe Nyssens and Bernadette Wynants (2001). "Modes d'organisation et dynamiques dans les services de proximité: vers un nouveau *welfare mix*?" in Jacques Defourny et al., *Économie sociale. Enjeux conceptuels, insertion par le travail et services de proximité*, Brussels, Éditions De Boeck Université.

Glazer, Nona (1993). *Women's Paid and Unpaid Labour: The Work Transfer in Health and Retailing*, Philadelphia, Temple University Press.

Glazer, Nona (1988). "Overlooked, Overworked: Women's Unpaid and Paid Work in the Health Services' 'Cost Crisis,'" *International Journal of Health Services*, 18:1, 119-137.

Godbout, Jacques (2000). *Le don, la dette et l'identité. Homo donator vs homo oeconomicus*, Montréal, Boréal.

Hollander, Marcus and Angela Tessaro (2001). *Evaluation of the Maintenance and Preventive Function of Home Care*, Ottawa, Home Care/Pharmaceuticals Division, Policy and Communication Branch, Health Canada.

Independent (2001). "CCAC needs more funds, says region," *New Hamburg Independent*, July 18.

James, Nicky (1989). "Emotional Labour: Skill and Work in the Social Regulation of Feelings," *Sociological Review*, 1, 15-42.

Laville, Jean-Louis (1994). "Économie et solidarité. Esquisse d'une problématique" in Laville, Jean-Louis (ed.), *L'Économie solidaire. Une perspective internationale*, Paris, Syros.

Laville, Jean-Louis (avec la collaboration de Rainer Duhm, Bernard Eme, Silvia Gherardi, Richard MacFarlane, Alan Thomas) (1993). *Les services de proximité en Europe. Pour une économie solidaire*, Paris, Syros/Alternatives.

Leira, Arnlaug (1994). "Concepts of Caring: Loving, Thinking, and Doing," *Social Service Review,* June, 185-201.

Leys, Colin (2001a). "The British National Health Service in the Face of Neo-Liberalism," in Pat Armstrong, Hugh Armstrong and David Coburn (eds.), *Unhealthy Times: Political Economy Perspectives on Health and Care in Canada*, Toronto, Oxford University Press, 66-90.

Leys, Colin (2001). *Market-driven Politics. Neoliberal Democracy and the Public Interest*, London, Verso.

Lukács, Georg (1980). *The Ontology of Social Being. 3. Labour*, translated by David Fernbach, London, Merlin.

Neysmith, Sheila M. (2000). "Networking Across Difference: Connecting Restructuring and Caring Labour," in Sheila Neysmith (ed.), *Restructuring Caring Labour: Discourse, State Practice, and Everyday Life*, Toronto, Oxford University Press.

Neysmith, Sheila M. (1998). "From Home Care to Social Care: The Value of a Vision," in Baines, Carol, Patricia Evans, Sheila Neysmith, *Women's Caring: Feminist Perspectives on Social Welfare,* second edition, Toronto, Oxford University Press, pp. 233-249.

Neysmith, Sheila & Jane Aronson (1997). "Working Conditions in Home Care: Negotiating Race and Class Boundaries in Gendered Work," *International Journal of Health Services*, 27:3, 479-499.

OCSA (2000). *Standards and Indicators for Personal Support & Homemaking Services*, Toronto, Ontario Community Support Association.

OCSA (1999). *Pre-Budget Consultation Submission to the Ontario Ministry of Finance*, Toronto, Ontario Community Support Association, April 1.

OHHCPA (1999). *Recruitment and Retention of the Home Care Sector Workforce*, Hamilton, Ontario Home Health Care Providers' Association.

Record (2001). "Empty beds at cancer hospice caused by cuts to home care," *Kitchener-Waterloo Record*, September 19.

Review (2001). "Health council keeping eye on CCAC cuts," *The Review* (Niagara Falls), July 19.

Saillant, Francine & Eric Gagnon, avec la collaboration de Catherine Montgomery, Steve Paquet et Robert Sévigny (2000). *De la dépendance et de l'accompagnement. Soins à domicile et liens sociaux*, Québec, L'Harmattan/Presses de l'Université Laval.

Shields, John & Evans, B. Mitchell (1998). *Shrinking the State: Globalization and Public Administration "Reform"*, Halifax, Fernwood Publishing.

Szasz, Andrew (1990). "The Labour Impacts of Policy Change in Health Care: How Federal Policy Transformed Home Health Organizations and Their Labour Practices," *Journal of Health Politics, Policy and Law*, 15:1.

Smith, Adam(1910). *An Enquiry into the Nature and Causes of the Wealth of Nations*, London, J.M. Dent.

Star (2001). "Cuts put 'people at risk': centre: Home care faces $1.9-M shortfall this year unless it makes `draconian' cuts to services," *The Sudbury Star*, July 4.

Twigg, Julia (2000a). *Bathing- the Body and Community Care*, London, Routledge.

Twigg, Julia (2000b). "Carework as a Form of Bodywork," *Ageing and Society*, 20, 389-411.

Weekly (2001). "VON feels effects of access cutbacks," *Northumberland Weekly*, July 20.

Whig Standard (2001a). "Access centre woes hit many communities," *Kingston Whig Standard*, September 29.

Whig Standard (2001b). "Providence cuts back, laying off 22," *The Kingston Whig-Standard*, July 6.

White, Jerry P. (1990). *Hospital Strike. Women, Unions, and Public Sector Conflict*, Toronto, Thompson Educational Publishing.

Williams, Allison (2001). "Home Care Restructuring at Work: The Impact of Policy Transformation on Women's Labour," in Isabel Dyck, Nancy Davis Lewis, and Sara McLafferty (eds.), *Geographies of Women's Health*, London, Routledge, 107-126.

Williams, Allison (1999). "An Assessment of Community Palliative Care Needs: The Case of Niagara," *Journal of Palliative Care*, 15:2, 45-52.

Williams, Allison, Michelle V. Caron, Maria McMillan, Anne Litkowich, Noreen Rutter, Arlete Hartman, John Yardley (2001). "An Evaluation of Contracted Palliative Care Home Care Services in Ontario, Canada," *Evaluation and Program Planning*, 24, 23-31.

Notes

[1] Earlier drafts of parts of this chapter were presented in May 2001 at the Congress of the Humanities and Social Sciences at Laval University, in June 2001 at the Tenth Canadian Social Welfare Policy Conference at the University of Calgary, in October 2001 at the conference on Community-based Organizations and the New Social Economy at the University of Regina, in March 2002 at Concordia University, in September 2002 at the Health and Human Rights Conference at Queen's University, and in June 2003 at the Congress of the Humanities and Social Sciences at Dalhousie University. My thanks to the organizers of, and participants in, those events. The research upon which this chapter is based was generously funded by Human Resources Development Canada under the *Économie sociale, santé et bien-être* project and by a strategic research grant from the Social Sciences and Humanities Research Council of Canada. I would like to thank Abdollah Payrow Shabani, David Welch, Gabriela Lopez, Marie-Ève Lavoie, and Pascale Houle for their assistance with various aspects of the research, and Michelle Weinroth, Phillip Hansen and Jane Aronson for reading earlier drafts of the paper.

[2] "In defining emotional labour as the labour involved in dealing with other people's feelings I am emphasizing that it is a social process. In noting that the regulation of emotion is a core component of emotional labour I am highlighting the centrality of the management of feelings within social processes."(James, 1989, 21)

[3] "To be effective the 'labourer's' skills must include firstly being able to understand and interpret the needs of others, secondly being able to provide a personal response to these needs, thirdly being able to juggle the delicate balance of each individual and of that individual within a group, and fourthly being able to pace the work, taking into account other responsibilities. Emotional labour requires learned skills in the same way that physical labour does. Access to the skills is open to anyone who has the interest or who has an obligation to learn them, but some practitioners are better than others. Like physical labour, there are certain techniques which, if adeptly applied, give a better outcome to emotional labour, both for the person caring

and for the person being cared for. In some circumstances, advice is sought, in others action is required, and in others a sense of perspective, of 'rightness,' is to be established." (James, 1989, 26)

4   "Finally, if relational services require 'co-production' by the provider and user, certain services are also responses to multi-dimensional demands, which require co-production by several different types of provider and hence the organization of an active personal relationship [*proximité active*] between them. Certain dependent, ill and/or isolated individuals, for example, need a combination of nursing, social, cleaning or friendly visiting services." (Gilain, Nyssens and Wynants, 2001, 92) See also Jean-Louis Laville's ideal-type of the solidarity-based economy, in which workers and users jointly produce the supply and demand of services, i.e. jointly work out what needs exist and how best to fulfil them. (Laville, 1994, 1993)

5   To be sure, by virtue of the division of labour, some caregivers have no physical relationship with those for whom they care. For example, volunteers who pay "friendly visits" to the frail elderly in their homes perform emotional labour, while, at the other end of the spectrum, a person sent by the Community Care Access Centre to install handles in a client's bathtub may perform only physical labour. The important thing to bear in mind, however, is that all of these labours are part of a continuum of care for the same individuals. The tasks only appear dissociated because of the division of labour between individuals, agencies and even government authorities.

6   "She told me in all seriousness that 'some shit don't stink.' I asked her to explain a bit more what she meant. As she was teaching me to make a bed, she made it perfectly clear: 'It depends on if you like 'em and they like you, and if you know them pretty well; it's hard to clean somebody new, or somebody you don't like. If you like them, it's like your baby.' A bit later she made reference to a man with whom she had had to struggle every day: 'But now take Floyd, that bastard, that man's shit is foul.' Through her explanation it became clear that the work is not a set of menial tasks, but a set of social relations in which the tasks are embedded." (T. Diamond, "Social Policy and Everyday Life in Nursing Homes: A Critical Ethnography," quoted by Twigg, 2000a, 153.)

7   "Le contact avec l'aidé, la possibilité d'établir un contact privilégié et singulier avec ce dernier, de recevoir son estime, sa reconnaissance, sont les aspects les plus appréciés dans les tâches, rémunérées ou non; et cela dans les trois milieux et chez toutes les catégories d'intervenantes. [...] Tout se passe à deux, dans une circulation de la reconnaissance de Soi et de l'Autre." (Saillant & Gagnon, 2000, 146-147)

8   This was said in the context of a seminar presentation at the University of Ottawa in February 2001.

9   But one ought to be careful about generalizations on this point, as there may be differences between families based on cultural factors.

10 "This suggests that the difficulty with intimate care is not simply one of incest but lies in a more generalized threat to the relationship. What is done is important here. The difficulty centres around tending what involves a diminution of the person—wiping their bottom, washing the body, feeding them—care that erodes their status as an adult. What older and disabled people dislike about intimate care is their loss of status in the eyes of the person who is close to them. They fear that the person they were—and to themselves still are—will be lost. Similarly carers want to continue to experience their mother/uncle/sister as the person they always knew, and that by and large functions and relates to them in a sociable way. It is a mistake to see intimacy as lying along a single continuum with strangers (least intimate) at one end and spouses (most intimate) at the other, and with physical and visual access graduated through. Though there is truth in this, it is too simple. Different sorts of intimacy pertain to different relationships.

"If kin relations can be problematic in this area, what about friends? Not surprisingly the same difficulties apply. Friendship classically rests on reciprocity and equality; and changes that disturb the equality, threaten the existence of the friendship. As a result, friendship is rarely the basis for caring in any long term or serious way; and this applies particularly in intimate care which transgresses the normal physical boundaries of friendship. [...]

"By general agreement, the preferred source of such care was a stranger, or at least someone who had started out as a stranger, but had then become familiar. What people wanted was a relationship with the careworker, but one that was specialized in nature, particular to the activity of caregiving, offering warmth and closeness, but within a defined and bounded set of expectations." (Twigg, 2000a, 73-74)

11 See Godbout (2000) on the difference between giving among kin and between non-kin.

12 "Furthermore, while trust is an issue common to all services—which are by their very nature 'experiential goods,' in the sense that their quality can only be grasped at the moment in which they are consumed—it is even more important in relational services (such as personal social services), the quality of which is intimately linked to the construction of the relationship between provider and user." (Gilain, Nyssens and Wynants, 2001, 91-92)

13 "Care managers purchase or allocate units of home care time at least as much as they allocate or purchase tasks. The privatization of care services and the purchaser/provider split have reinforced this tendency. Staff in care agencies increasingly work to time schedules that specify the time each task should take and the point at which they should move to their next client."(Twigg, 2000a, 99)

14   "While not all emotional labour is carried out by women, it builds on skills women learn as part of what Oakley refers to as their 'long apprenticeship.' (Oakley, 1974) With new systems of scientific management being implemented, and management accountability at a premium (see Griffiths Report, 1984) it is hard to imagine where the work carried out by emotional labourers will fit in. Since the work is rarely recognized, management methods of accounting for it are even rarer, and where they exist at all they are in their infancy. Yet this does not detract from the evidence that such work is done in the public sector, in industry and commerce, and will continue to need to be done."(James, 1989, 37)

15   "We feel guilty when we leave a day's work. We were nurses and practical nurses. We did it all. We haven't been able to be as caring as we used to be... There is simply no time to sit with dying patients so they die alone." (Nurse quoted by Laura Sky, *Lean and Mean Health Care*, cited in Armstrong et al., 1997, 144.)

16   "Above all, the close interpersonal nature of bodycare means that the principles of efficiency and of care are in conflict to a significant degree. Efficiency suggests that production should follow the model of MacDonald's with an emphasis on repeateability, on efficiencies of scale, of standardized interactions and limited involvement, but 'care' is structured differently. Care requires that the response be highly individual, specific to that person and to that moment. It is by its nature interactive, forged at the front line and cannot be separated from that setting or that interaction. Its remit is also unbounded, resting as it does on a response to the needs of the person as a whole rather than specific and localized care deficits. Care rests on an unbounded ethic that is in conflict with the focussed, instrumental nature of waged work..."(Twigg, 2000a, 122)

17   "[Schweikhart and Smith-Daniels] categorize nursing work as being either *care production* or *care management* tasks, although they note that there may be some overlaps between the two. Care production, they say 'represents the hands-on execution of each patient's care plan' that 'tends to be highly-structured, task-oriented and repetitive' such as 'assisting patients with activities for daily living, monitoring of vital signs, administering IVs, medications, and treatments and giving patient and family education.' 'Care management is concerned with planning and coordinating care delivery activities [...] and is typically characterized by relatively high levels of decision-making, autonomy and accountability.' This work 'directly includes communication and coordination among clinicians and other care providers and indirectly helps advance the clinical expertise of staff and the knowledge base of the organization.'" (Campbell, 2000, 191)

18   "'The director of nursing has said ... [we] need to revamp our thinking. They don't need a bath every day. They don't need their linen changed every day..' This type of undermining of what the health care worker be-

lieves to be real care can lead to stress and a reduction in the attachment to work." (Armstrong et al., *Voices from the Ward*, in Armstrong et al., 1997, 145)

[19] For analyses of commodification in the British National Health Service that in many ways parallel this, see Colin Leys (2001).

[20] See Williams (1999) and Williams et al. (2001) for accounts of how CCACs have attempted to evaluate the services they purchase.

[21] "Rather this is a sector that had traditionally relied on naturalized concepts of good practice. Thus good home care helps are so because they are naturally caring people. Careworkers can be relied upon to respond well to clients because of the sorts of people they are, not because of any customer training they have gone through. This both reinforces the ideal of authenticity—they are nice because they *are* nice—at the same time as undercutting any claims that might be made for better pay or conditions on the basis of qualifications."(Twigg, 2000a, 121)

[22] Saillant and Gagnon interestingly relate the overriding need for trust and authenticity in the care relationship to the blurring of kinship structures. The roles and expectations between parents and adult children are no longer set but, to a much greater extent than previously, freely chosen. The resulting uncertainty is very destabilizing. In the absence of stable ties, the establishment of equitably and freely constituted relations is crucial. Authentic speech and disinterested acts are the new foundation of such relations. Speech in itself is the purpose sought in some care relationships (e.g., friendly visiting), and it is at the heart even of those that seem to consist merely in material services, such as house cleaning. (Saillant & Gagnon, 2000, 204)

[23] "In Hochschild's account, emotional labour is damaging to the workers because it erodes authenticity and, through the deep acting it requires, corrupts the capacity to feel. This was not how the careworkers in the study perceived things. Though caring could be emotionally tiring, particularly for a demanding or depressed client, the danger of the work came not from self-estrangement, but from the reality and strength of the ties that it created. Getting attached to clients was an occupational hazard as well as a source of pleasure. Strong feelings were inevitable, particularly where contact was sustained."(Twigg, 2000a, 166) "The most successful workers (and they included some whose caring was highly commended by both clients and managers) were those who could switch off their emotions once they had left."(Twigg, 2000a, 167)

[24] As Marie Campbell puts it, with reference to hospital work: "When managerial technologies—not individual nurses—plan the work, the hospital's need to reduce expenditures on non-value-added work appears to be accommodated. In managerial texts, the nurse as active subject is lost sight of in the shift of authority that takes place when nursing decisions are preplanned and reassigned away from her, but there is a wild card in this

otherwise tidy organizational process. In actual health care workplaces, unexpected things happen that continually require reliably intelligent intervention by nurses. No plan can be counted on exclusively because, as Jackson observed, no plan ever 'gets it right.' The eliminated nurse is constantly being expected to hold nursing workplaces together, but she has to do so behind the scenes in an unrecognized way. This is what I call the virtually disappeared nurse." (2000, 193) This is arguably true in every workplace subjected to hierarchical authority and bureaucratic rationalization. Hence the threatening nature of work-to-rule campaigns. See Browne (1992) on how the discrepancy between the abstract plan and the concrete reality breeds crises.

25 "In these circumstances, the nurses accept a commonsense understanding of 'work' as 'doing something,' physical work, thus excluding emotional labour from their definitions of work. The insidious effect of pressure to 'work' is that tasks gradually become pre-eminent, and then other work, such as emotional labour, is carried out as 'time' allows. From being a part of a 'whole,' gradually, through the circumstances in which it is carried out, the psycho-social work becomes secondary."(James, 1989, 35)

26 See Saillant & Gagnon (2000, 107) on the importance of time and rituals in carework.

27 "[Emotional labour] is recognized not when the outcome is right, but on those occasions when it goes wrong. The product itself is invisible. The value of the labour is only recognized in negative forms, in disorder, rather than in its positive form of 'adjustment.' So for the main part the value of the labour is as hidden as the value of the routine management of emotion."(James, 1989, 28)

28 "...though you may schedule a period of time in which to do the task, its accomplishment is never certain, so the time of carework and the time of clock work are never quite the same. This applies both to the bodywork element in care: the constant entropy of leaking bodies; and the emotional dimension. Careworkers find it hard to leave clients who are distressed and need them at that moment. Putting limits on the work whether in terms of time and emotion is often hard; and there is an essentially unbounded character to care." (Twigg, 2000a, 172)

29 "Emotional labour is most easily recognized as part of the caring role of women in the home. Although the social regulation of emotions is brought about through emotional labour, as a form of labour it appears to be insulated from other forms of labour, and is poorly recorded and under-explored. It is my contention that this is precisely because it involves both women and 'emotion,' with their negative connotations. Because emotional labour is seen as 'natural,' unskilled women's work, because it is unpaid and because it is obscured by the privacy of the domestic domain where much of it takes place, the significance of its contribution and value in social

reproduction is ignored.[...] Thus the supposed 'naturalness' of women's caring role is central to the significance, value and invisibility of emotional labour and its development through gender identity and work roles. Part of women's caring role is that they are deemed to be 'naturally' good at dealing with other people's emotions because they are themselves 'naturally' emotional—though this does also mean that they are also unreliable." (James, 1989, 22)

30 Thus, in defining standards for home care services, the Ontario Community Support Association ranks continuity among eight criteria of quality: "Standards under each quality responsibility areas were organized by eight measurable dimensions of quality: safety, provider competence, acceptability, accessibility, efficiency, appropriateness, effectiveness and continuity. The first seven measurable dimensions of quality have been used and published extensively in quality improvement literature. These dimensions identify the key elements of quality services. The [Canadian Council on Health Services Accreditation] incorporated these dimensions in their Standards for Accreditation and added another dimension, continuity. Continuity has been included in these standards because of its importance to personal support and homemaking services in the community." (OCSA, 2000, 4)

31 This was made clear to me in interviews with the directors of agencies which had won and lost CCAC contracts.

32 "I think we lost a control thing, though (and I think that did have a lot to do with managed competition), because we get paid per visit, so if the nurses aren't out doing visits, they're not generating money. So how can you bring them in twice a week for two hours and have them sitting here doing work that could be done by office staff? In order to keep us out in the district seeing more patients, doing visits, generating income, they've got these non-nurses planning our work for us and that's where we lost control." (Interview with Ottawa home care nurse, November 2000.) "...we used to have local offices in little communities (...) They were fully staffed offices with a nurse manager, but we consolidated all our caseload planning and computerized it, so it's all in one location now. So we reduced our management time, which I think we had to do anyway, but it has meant that the staff sometimes feel that they don't have the support when they go into the field. Two years ago they could drop into the office at the end of the day and talk about problems. Today, they have to do it over the phone and they don't do it to the same degree obviously." (Interview with director of home care agency, February 2001.)

Contributors

Pat Armstrong, Ph.D., is co-author of such books on health care as *Heal Thyself: Managing Health Care Reform*; *Wasting Away: The Undermining of Canadian Health Care*; *Universal Health Care: What the United States Can Learn From Canada*; *Vital Signs: Nursing in Transition;* and *Take Care: Warning Signals for Canada's Health System*. She has also published on a wide variety of issues related to women's work and social policy. She has served as Chair of the Department of Sociology at York University and Director of the School of Canadian Studies at Carleton University. She is a partner in the National Network on Environments and Women's Health and chairs a working group on health reform that crosses the Centres of Excellence for Women's Health. Her current SSHRC-funded research compares care management in Canada and the United States. Like most of her past research, this project relies primarily on the perspectives of those who actually provide or manage care within the system. She holds a CHSRF/CIHR Chair in Health Services.

Paul Leduc Browne, D.Phil., is an associate professor of political science at the Université du Québec en Outaouais. He was previously a research fellow with the Canadian Centre for Policy Alternatives for eight years. His fields of expertise are health and social policy, with a specific focus on home care and the non-profit sector. He is the author of *Unsafe Practices: Restructuring and Privatization in Ontario Health Care* (CCPA Books, 2000) and *Love in a Cold World? The Voluntary Sector in an Age of Cuts* (CCPA Books, 1996), and co-editor with Douglas Moggach of *The Social Question and the Democratic Revolution* (University of Ottawa Press, 2000).

Tamara Daly is a Canadian Health Services Research Foundation postdoctoral fellow at the Centre for Health Studies at York University. She received her Ph.D. in health policy from the University of Toronto and holds a Master of Arts in political economy from Carleton

University. Her Ph.D. thesis focused on the impact of funding changes on non-profit organizations that provide home health and social care.

Olga Kits received her M.A. from Queen's University specializing in social theory, philosophy and sociology of science, and medical sociology. She has previously participated in a variety of research projects with organizations such as Health Canada's Canadian Cancer Control Strategy, International Centre for the Advancement of Community Based Rehabilitation (Centre of Excellence), National Cancer Institute of Canada, and the Canadian Cancer Society.

Denise O'Connor is a Ph.D. Candidate at McMaster University (Comparative Public Policy). She is studying the role of power and ideology in the home-care policy communities of Ontario and Britain, and their effect on the capacity of local organizations to deliver home-care services effectively. Her interest in home care emerged from her exposure to the effect of managed competition during her six-year tenure as a volunteer board member for a large, non-profit homemaking organization in Hamilton.

Allison Williams, Ph.D., is a research professor with the Saskatchewan Population Health and Evaluation Research Unit (SPHERU) and an Assistant Professor in the Department of Geography at the University of Saskatchewan. She is active in investigating the relations between health and the environment from a geographical perspective, with a particular focus on the concept of therapeutic landscapes, which holistically grasps ways in which environments operate as determinants of and pathways to health. She is involved in several partnerships with public-health departments, community groups and various health-care organizations. She was recently awarded a New Investigator Career Award by the Canadian Institutes for Health Research.